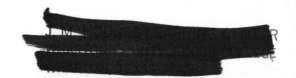

# THE COMPREHENSIVE
# DIABETIC COOKBOOK

# THE COMPREHENSIVE

# DIABETIC COOKBOOK

by

## DOROTHY J. KAPLAN

WITH A FOREWORD BY

*Robert Kaye, M.D.*

Head of Diabetic Clinic, Children's

Hospital of Philadelphia

FREDERICK FELL, INC.　　*New York*

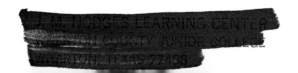

*For information address:*
Frederick Fell, Inc.
386 Park Avenue South
New York, N.Y. 10016

Library of Congress Catalog Card No. 70-108032

*Published simultaneously in Canada by*
George J. McLeod, Limited, Toronto 2B, Ontario

Manufactured in the United States of America

Standard Book Number 8119-0191-2

# Foreword

Mrs. Kaplan has very successfully managed all aspects of diabetic regulation since her daughter became diabetic at the age of two years.

I believe that her manual offers a great deal which will be useful to other diabetics and to individuals interested in controlling or reducing their weight. The scope of the manual is so extensive that the user will be enabled to enjoy a widely varied diet without sacrificing accurate control of calories and composition. Presentation of individual food items in terms of calories, protein, carbohydrate, and fat composition as well as in the exchange system is particularly helpful to users who may be familiar with only one or the other system of calculation.

In addition, the manual will be a valuable adjunct to the doctor and will satisfy a need which I have long felt in my practice with reference to children with diabetes and obesity. I, for one, am grateful to Mrs. Kaplan for having taken the great pains to bring this comprehensive book to completion.

ROBERT KAYE, M.D.
*Professor of Pediatrics*
University of Pennsylvania
School of Medicine
Children's Hospital of
Philadelphia

# Contents

# Introduction

Since our daughter developed diabetes, I have spent a great deal of time calculating and revising our favorite recipes, developing new ones, and writing to companies to acquire carbohydrate, protein, and fat breakdowns of their products. Having this information greatly simplified my menu planning. As the diabetic diet is a natural, well-balanced one, I preferred making the same dishes for the entire family to cooking two separate meals three times a day. It was a challenge to make our meals interesting, varied, and delicious.

The result of this research and investigation was the compilation of this "manual." And once it took shape, grew, and I began using it, I realized how handy and timesaving it was. I hope that other diabetics, those cooking for diabetics, and those interested in wholesome, tasty recipes will find it of help.

The diabetic's diet must be carefully balanced in carbohydrates, proteins, and fat; the exchange system enables this balance to be maintained easily. Your physician will work out your menus by calculating how many exchanges you are allowed per meal in every category. Using this manual you can then plan varied and delicious meals. Suppose he tells you your breakfast should consist of:

1 fruit exchange
1½ bread exchanges
2 meat exchanges
½ milk exchange
1 fat exchange

Turning to the fruit section of this manual you can see that you might have ½ cup orange juice *or* 1 orange *or* 1 peach *or* ½ banana *or* any other listing under fruit exchange. Your 1½ bread exchanges might be ¾ cup dry cereal (1 bread exchange) and ½ piece toast (½ bread exchange) *or* 1½ pieces toast (1½ bread exchanges) *or* 1½ muffins (1½ bread exchanges) *or* any other total of 1½ under the bread exchange. Your 2 meat exchanges could be 2 scrambled eggs (or poached or soft boiled, etc.) *or* 2 ounces of meat. The ½ milk exchange, which would be 4 ounces of whole milk, could be used in your cereal. The one fat exchange could be a slice of bacon to go with your eggs *or* 1 teaspoon of butter or margarine to go on your toast. (If you used skim milk instead of whole milk, you would have an additional fat exchange and then have two slices of bacon *or* 1 slice of bacon and 1 teaspoon of butter or margarine because this additional fat exchange would give you a total of 2.)

If your diet is set up in calories, rather than exchanges, follow the same procedure using the calorie listing under each exchange:

> 1 milk exchange—170 calories
> 1 vegetable B exchange—36 calories
> 1 fruit exchange—40 calories
> 1 bread exchange—68 calories
> 1 meat exchange—73 calories
> 1 fat exchange—45 calories

Many diabetics have followed this system for years but were unable to eat anything other than those foods listed in each exchange category. They were not able to eat a mixed food, such as meat loaf or potato salad or chicken cacciatora or any recipe that called for a combination of ingredients because they couldn't figure out how much of each exchange the serving of food would provide. Here we provide the answer to this problem. Every recipe in this book lists the exchanges that a serving will provide. If you have a serving of potato salad in Chapter V, you will know that you are consuming one bread exchange and four fat exchanges. One serving of ribbon meat loaf in Chapter IX will provide you with three meat exchanges, one bread exchange and one fat exchange. You can see immediately how much of each dish the diabetic may eat using the diet outlined by your physician. Everyone will benefit; the diabetic will eat tasty dishes and the rest of the family will eat the well-balanced meals on which all diabetic diets are based.

Thus, you can see the value and outstanding merit of this system. There is great variety of meal-planning and ease of cooking because the exchange system and these recipes are based on handy household measures. In addition, after you have become familiar with these recipes, you can turn to the appendix and, using the forms provided, calculate your own favorite dishes.

The emphasis on dietary control of diabetes is being stressed more today than ever before, and a proper diet that is tasty and easy to follow is as important as the medication prescribed. My sincere hope is that the recipes in this book will make it easier for you to follow the proper diet, and that this will add happy and healthy years to your life.

DJK

# To the Weight Watcher

There are very few people who haven't tried a "fad" or "crash" diet once or twice, knowing that the real answer to losing weight and maintaining the proper scale-reading is sensible, well-balanced, controlled eating. The diabetic formula can easily be adapted by the normal weight watcher.

The first step is a visit to your physician. After a checkup and discussion as to your weight requirements, he will work out for you a diet based on exchanges; you will know how much of each exchange you are allowed per meal and thus, using his list and this manual as a guide, you can plan your daily meals. They will be adequate, varied, interesting, and calculated for you, so your eating program will be well-balanced and you will be on your way to your proper weight.

For instance, let us say your doctor prescribes the following 1500-calorie-per-day diet for you:

*Breakfast*

1 fruit exchange
1 meat exchange
1 bread exchange
1 fat exchange
½ milk exchange

*Lunch*

3 meat exchanges
1 veg. A exchange
1 veg. B exchange
1½ bread exchanges
2 fat exchanges
1 fruit exchange
½ milk exchange

*Dinner*

3 meat exchanges
1 veg. A exchange
1 veg. B exchange
1 bread exchange
1 fat exchange
1 fruit exchange
½ milk exchange

*Snack*

½ milk exchange
1 bread exchange

Using the exchange lists at the head of each of the seven categories—milk, vegetable A, vegetable B, fruit, bread, meat, fat—and adding the calculated recipes in this manual, you can plan countless different meals. For dinner you could have:

Flank steak
Pseudo sweet-potato casserole
Cauliflower with ½ teaspoon margarine
1 apple muffin with ½ teaspoon margarine
Jellied blanc mange with 2 cinnamon cookies

OR

½ fruit cocktail (water pack) on ⅛ cup sherbet (made with water)
Ribbon meat loaf
½ cup beets
Lettuce and tomato salad
Pudding surprise

OR

Barbecued chuck roast
Baked potato with ½ teaspoon margarine
Broccoli
1 quick blender popover
Cherry cream pie in rice crispy crust

As you can see, the possibilities are endless and the results truly delicious.

In planning a meal, list the exchanges allowed for that meal. Then, as you select a recipe and see what exchanges will be used in a serving, cross out those exchanges on your list. In that manner you can see what you have left as you go along. Be sure to carefully measure each serving.

Following this system is like playing a game; you will come up with different, delicious meals all the time and you won't believe you're weight-watching!

### A Special Note Regarding "Dietetic" or "Sugar-Free" Packaged Foods

It is most important to realize that all foods must be calculated in the diet. If something says "dietetic" or "sugar-free," it still has calories and must be counted. Most of these special foods have a substance called "sorbitol" substituted for sugar and it is stated that this substance is utilized by the body at a much slower rate than sugar would be utilized. This is true, but since the substance is utilized by the body, the calories must be subtracted from the daily allowance. All such special products state the caloric content on the container. It is wise to compare the calories in the artificially sweetened product with the real thing. Often the difference is negligible and the dietetic or sugar-free product does not usually taste as good. If you have to count the calories anyway, why not enjoy the better flavor.

# THE COMPREHENSIVE
# DIABETIC COOKBOOK

# CHAPTER I

# Milk

## MILK EXCHANGES

*One milk exchange consists of:*

| | |
|---|---|
| Carbohydrate | 12 gm. |
| Protein | 8 gm. |
| Fat | 10 gm. |
| Calories | 170 |

The following each equal 1 milk exchange:

| | |
|---|---|
| Whole milk | 1 cup |
| Evaporated milk | ½ cup |
| Powdered milk | ¼ cup |
| Buttermilk | 1 cup |
| Skim milk * | 1 cup |
| Yogurt † | 1 cup |

Dessert and beverage recipes sometimes provide milk exchanges. If you will refer to Chapter XVII you will find the following recipes can be figured in your diet as milk exchanges:

Cherry Cream Pie Filling
Baked Custard
Jellied Blanc Mange
Baked Alaska
Pudding Surprize
Parfait Royale

In Chapter XX, Beverages, you will find a recipe for Milkshakes that is calculated in Milk Exchanges.

* Add two fat exchanges if nonfat milk is used
† Add one fat exchange

# CHAPTER II

# Vegetable A

## VEGETABLE A

| | | |
|---|---|---|
| Carbohydrate | gm. | |
| Protein | gm. | Negligible amounts in |
| Fat | gm. | 1-cup servings |
| Calories | | |

Asparagus
Broccoli
Brussel sprouts
Cabbage
Cauliflower
Celery
Chicory
Cucumber
Escarole
Eggplant
Lettuce
Endive
Beet greens
Mustard greens
Turnip greens
Spinach
Chard
Collard
Dandelion greens
Kale
Tomatoes
Mushrooms
Okra
Peppers
Radishes
Rhubarb
Sauerkraut

Young string beans
Summer squash
Parsley

Frozen vegetables cooked in butter sauce—add 1 fat exchange for each ½ cup serving.

Frozen vegetables can be baked. Place block in casserole; spread with margarine, sprinkle with salt (for limas only, add ¼ cup water). Cover and bake along with dinner. (Be sure to calculate margarine out of fat allowance.)

Chart is for baking at 350 degrees. If baking at 325 degrees increase time ten minutes; if baking at 375 degrees decrease time ten minutes.

40 to 50 minutes

Broccoli
Peas
Spinach
Squash
Brussels sprouts
Whole kernel corn
Limas, large

50 to 60 minutes

Asparagus
Cauliflower
Green beans
Limas, small
Mixed vegetables
Peas and carrots
Succotash

RECIPE FOR

# Fabulous Salad

| Ingredients | Measure | Carbohydrates (gm.) | Protein (gm.) | Fat (gm.) |
|---|---|---|---|---|
| Eggplant, medium, cubed | 1 | | | |
| Zucchini, medium, sliced | 3 | 6 | 1 | |
| Green pepper, cubed | 2 | | | |
| Tomatoes, cubed | 2 | | | |
| Onions, sliced, large | 3 | 21 | 6 | |
| Garlic, sliced | 2 | | | |
| Mushrooms, sliced | 1 pound | | | |
| Oil | ¼ cup | | | 60 |
| Tomato juice | ½ cup | | | |
| Salt | 2 teaspoons | | | |
| Pepper | ½ teaspoon | | | |
| | | 27 | 7 | 60 |

Calories: 1 serving—67.6     2.7  .7  6

Combine all ingredients in large baking dish, season with salt and pepper and mix well. Bake 40 minutes at 350°. Stir once or twice.

Servings: 10
Exchange per serving: 1½ fat

# Smothered Onions

| Ingredients | Measure | Car-bohy-drates (gm.) | Pro-tein (gm.) | Fat (gm.) |
|---|---|---|---|---|
| Margarine | ¼ cup | | | 60 |
| Onions, peeled and thinly sliced | 10 medium | 28 | 8 | |
| Salt | 1 teaspoon | | | |
| Pepper | ⅛ teaspoon | | | |
| Worcestershire sauce | 2 teaspoons | | | |
| Liquid hot pepper seasoning | dash | | | |
| | | 28 | 8 | 60 |
| Calories: 1 serving—68.4 | | 2.8 | .8 | 6 |

Slowly heat margarine in large skillet. Add rest of ingredients. Cook, over low heat and stirring occasionally, 30 minutes or until onions are nicely browned.

Servings: 10
Exchange per serving: 1 fat

# Zing Salad

| Ingredients | Measure | Carbohydrates (gm.) | Protein (gm.) | Fat (gm.) |
|---|---|---|---|---|
| Green beans, drained | 2 cups | | | |
| Carrots, sliced and drained | 2 cups | 28 | 8 | |
| Kidney beans, drained | 2 cups | 79.2 | 29.2 | 2 |
| Onion, sliced | 1 small | 7 | 2 | |
| Green pepper, chopped | ¼ cup | | | |
| Celery, chopped | ¼ cup | | | |
| Parsley | 2 tablespoons | | | |
| White vinegar | ½ cup | | | |
| Artificial sweetener | = ½ cup sugar | | | |
| Salad oil | 2 tablespoons | | | 30 |
| Salt | 1 teaspoon | | | |
| Dry mustard | 1 teaspoon | | | |
| | | 114.2 | 39.2 | 32 |

Calories: 1 serving—88.6

11.4  4  3

Place first 7 ingredients in shallow dish. In separate container, with tight lid, place next 5 ingredients. Shake well. Pour over vegetables and refrigerate overnight.

Servings: 10
Exchange per serving: 1 bread, ½ fat

# Escalloped Tomatoes

| Ingredients | Measure | Carbohydrates (gm.) | Protein (gm.) | Fat (gm.) |
|---|---|---|---|---|
| Onion, chopped | 3 tablespoons | | | |
| Margarine, melted | 1 tablespoon | | | 15 |
| Tomatoes | 2 16-ounce cans | | | |
| Artificial sweetener | = ½ teaspoon sugar | | | |
| Salt | ¾ teaspoon | | | |
| Pepper | ½ teaspoon | | | |
| Soft bread crumbs, toasted | 1½ cups | 45 | 6 | |
| | | 45 | 6 | 15 |
| Calories: 1 serving—118.3 | | 11.2 | 1.5 | 3.7 |

Sauté onion in margarine until tender. Add tomatoes, artificial sweetener, salt, and pepper; turn into 1-quart casserole. Top with bread crumbs. Bake at 375 degrees for 20 minutes. Stir lightly and serve.

Servings: 4
Exchange per serving: 1 fruit, 1 fat

# Tomatoes Provencal

| Ingredients | Measure | Car-bohy-drates (gm.) | Pro-tein (gm.) | Fat (gm.) |
|---|---|---|---|---|
| Tomatoes | 6 large | | | |
| Salt | as desired | | | |
| Pepper | as desired | | | |
| Fresh bread crumbs | 1 cup | 30 | 4 | |
| Finely chopped parsley | 2 tablespoons | | | |
| Olive oil | 1 teaspoon | | | 5 |
| | | 30 | 4 | 5 |

Calories: 1 serving—29.6      5    .6    .8

    Wash tomatoes and cut in half, crosswise. Place halves, cut side up, in shallow baking pan. Sprinkle each lightly with salt and pepper. Combine bread crumbs and parsley. Sprinkle over surface of tomato halves. Sprinkle each lightly with olive oil; bake at 450 degrees for 10 to 15 minutes or until golden brown on top.

Servings: 6
Exchange per serving: ½ fruit

# Pickles

| Ingredients | Measure | Car-bohy-drates (gm.) | Pro-tein (gm.) | Fat (gm.) |
|---|---|---|---|---|
| Small, hard pickling cucumbers | ½ bushel | | | |
| Salt | 1 tablespoon per jar | | | |
| Garlic, diced | 1 clove per jar | | | |
| Pickling spice | ¼ teaspoon per jar | | | |
| Dill flower | 2 per jar | | | |

Scrub cucumbers with sponge or brush. Pack tightly in clean quart jars. Add remaining ingredients. Fill each jar to top with cold water. Use two-piece metal tops; boil tops and put on jars when hot; tighten and turn upside down for 24 hours. Check for leakage. Turn right side up and store in cool dark place. Ready in approximately 3 weeks. Will keep indefinitely until opened.

Can pickle tomatoes the same way by substituting hard, green tomatoes for the pickles and one half stalk celery for the two dill flowers.

Servings: 20 to 24 jars
Exchange per serving: free

# CHAPTER III

# Vegetable B

## VEGETABLE B

| | |
|---|---|
| Carbohydrate | 7 gm. |
| Protein | 2 gm. |
| Calories | 36 |

Beets
Carrots
Onions
Green peas
Pumpkin
Rutabaga
Winter squash
Turnips
Mixed vegetables

Vegetables frozen in butter sauce—add 1 fat exchange per ½ cup serving.

# Green Bean Casserole

| Ingredients | Measure | Carbohydrates (gm.) | Protein (gm.) | Fat (gm.) |
|---|---|---|---|---|
| Cream of chicken soup | 1 10½-ounce can | 20.7 | 9.6 | 17.4 |
| Soy sauce | 1 teaspoon | | | |
| French fried onion rings | 3 ounces | 22 | 3 | 15 |
| French style green beans, cooked | 2 1-pound cans, drained | | | |
| Pepper | dash | | | |
| | | 42.7 | 12.6 | 32.4 |
| Calories: 1 serving—85.4 | | 7.1 | 2.1 | 5.4 |

In a 1-quart casserole stir soup and soy sauce until smooth; mix in half the onions, all the beans, and the pepper. Bake at 350 degrees for 20 minutes or until bubbling. Top with remaining onions. Bake 5 minutes more.

Servings: 6
Exchange per serving: 1 vegetable B, 1 fat

# Carrot Pennies

| Ingredients | Measure | Car-bohy-drates (gm.) | Pro-tein (gm.) | Fat (gm.) |
|---|---|---|---|---|
| Carrots, very thinly sliced | 1 quart | 56 | 16 | |
| Dried basil leaves | ½ teaspoon | | | |
| Salt | ½ teaspoon | | | |
| Pepper | few grains | | | |
| Water | ¼ cup | | | |
| Margarine | 2 tablespoons | | | 30 |
| | | 56 | 16 | 30 |

Calories: 1 serving—92.6          9.3   2.6   5

Place carrots in 1½-quart casserole. Sprinkle with basil, salt, and pepper; toss together. Add water and dot with margarine. Cover and bake at 350 degrees for 65 to 70 minutes, until fork tender.

Servings: 6
Exchange per serving: 1 vegetable B, 1 fat

# Pseudo Sweet-Potato Casserole

| Ingredients | Measure | Carbohydrates (gm.) | Protein (gm.) | Fat (gm.) |
|---|---|---|---|---|
| Frozen squash, mashed | 2 packages | 72.8 | 11.2 | 3.2 |
| Artificial sweetener | = 18 teaspoons sugar | | | |
| Maple flavoring, dietetic | ½ teaspoon | | | |
| Dietetic orange marmalade | ¼ cup | | | |
| Brown sugar | 2 tablespoon | 26 | | |
| Cinnamon | 1 teaspoon | | | |
| Salt | 1 teaspoon | | | |
| | | 98.8 | 11.2 | 3.2 |

Calories: 1 serving—58.4

|  | 12.3 | 1.4 | .4 |
|---|---|---|---|

Thaw frozen squash in top of double boiler. Combine with all other ingredients. Stir until well blended. Pour into lightly oiled casserole. Bake at 350 degrees for 30 minutes.

Servings: 8
Exchange per serving: 1 vegetable B, ½ fruit

# Orange Squash

| Ingredients | Measure | Carbohydrates (gm.) | Protein (gm.) | Fat (gm.) |
|---|---|---|---|---|
| Frozen squash, thawed | 2 packages | 72.8 | 11.2 | 3.2 |
| Margarine | ¼ cup | | | 60 |
| Brown sugar | 4 tablespoons | 26 | | |
| Orange juice | ¼ cup | 5 | | |
| Salt | 1 teaspoon | | | |
| Pepper | Dash | | | |
| Orange rind, grated | 1 tablespoon | | | |
| | | 103.8 | 11.2 | 63.2 |
| Calories: 1 serving—129.6 | | 13 | 1.4 | 8 |

Combine ingredients in top of double boiler. Heat until hot and bubbly.

Servings: 8
Exchange per serving: 1 bread, 1½ fat

# CHAPTER IV

# Fruit

FRUIT

Carbohydrate    10 gm.
Calories    40

| | |
|---|---|
| Apple | 1 small (2-inch diameter) |
| Applesauce | ½ cup |
| Apricots, fresh | 2 medium |
| Apricots, dried | 4 halves |
| Banana | ½ small |
| Berries (strawberries, raspberries, or blackberries) | 1 cup |
| Blueberries | ⅔ cup |
| Cantaloupe | ¼ (6-inch diameter) |
| Cherries | 10 large |
| Dates | 2 |
| Figs, fresh | 2 large |
| Figs, dried | 1 small |
| Fruit cup | ½ cup |
| Grapefruit | ½ small |
| Grapes | 12 |
| Honeydew | ⅛ (7-inch diameter) |
| Ice or sherbet, without milk | ¼ cup |
| Jelly | 2 teaspoons |
| Mango | ½ small |
| Orange | 1 small |
| Papaya | ⅓ medium |
| Peach | 1 medium |
| Pear | 1 small |
| Pineapple | 1 slice or ½ cup |
| Plums | 2 medium |
| Prunes, dried | 2 medium |
| Raisins | 2 tablespoons |
| Sugar | 2 teaspoons |

| Tangerine | 1 large |
| Watermelon | 1 cup |
| Maraschino cherries | 2 |

## JUICES

| Cranberry | ⅓ cup |
| Grape | ¼ cup |
| Orange, grapefruit | ½ cup |
| Pineapple, apple, prune | ⅓ cup |
| Gingerale | ½ cup |

## BIRD'S EYE FRUIT

| ¼ package melon balls (4 ounces) | 1 fruit |
| ⅓ package mixed fruit (4 ounces) | 3 fruit |
| ⅓ cup peaches (4 ounces) | 2½ fruit |
| ½ cup strawberry halves (5 ounces) | 4 fruit |
| ⅔ cup whole strawberries (5 ounces) | 3 fruit |

## BIRD'S EYE JUICES

| 4 ounces Awake | 1⅓ fruit |
| 4 ounces grapefruit juice | 1⅓ fruit |
| 4 ounces limeade | 1⅓ fruit |
| 4 ounces orange juice | 1⅓ fruit |
| 4 ounces orange-grapefruit juice | 1⅓ fruit |
| 4 ounces pink lemonade | 1⅓ fruit |
| 4 ounces lemonade | 1⅓ fruit |
| 1 Mrs. Paul's Apple Fritters | 1 fruit |

Many dessert recipes provide fruit exchanges. If you will refer to Chapter XVII, you will find the following recipes can be figured in your diet as fruit exchanges:

Apple Torte
Graham Cracker Crust
Rice Crispy Cereal Crust
Cool la la Lime Pie Filling

Cherry Cream Pie Filling
Fruit Whip
Hawaiian Dessert
Strawberry Whip
Eclairs
Baked Alaska
Parfait Royale

# Gelatin and Fruit Salad

| Ingredients | Measure | Carbohydrates (gm.) | Protein (gm.) | Fat (gm.) |
|---|---|---|---|---|
| Dietetic gelatin | 1 envelope | | | |
| Water | 1 cup | | | |
| Fruit | 2 exchanges | 20 | | |
| Lettuce | 2 leaves | | | |
| | | 20 | | |
| Calories: 1 serving—40 | | 10 | | |

Prepare gelatin according to package directions. Pour into 2 individual ring molds and chill until firm. Unmold onto lettuce and fill with 1 fruit exchange each: ½ diced banana; ½ chopped apple, sprinkled with cinnamon; ½ cup cubed pineapple.

Servings: 2
Exchange per serving: 1 fruit

# CHAPTER V

# Bread

## BREAD

| Carbohydrate | 15 gm. |
|---|---|
| Protein | 2 gm. |
| Calories | 68 |

| | |
|---|---|
| Bagel | ½ |
| Bread (white, whole wheat, rye) | 1 slice |
| Hollywood | 2 slices |
| Biscuit, roll, muffin | 1 (2-inch diameter) |
| Cornbread | 1 (1½-inch cube) |
| Flour | 2½ tablespoons |
| Cornstarch | 2 tablespoons |
| Tapioca, dry | 2 tablespoons |
| Cereal, cooked | ½ cup |
| Cereal, dry | ¾ cup |
| Rice, grits—cooked | ½ cup |
| Spaghetti, noodles, macaroni | ½ cup |
| Crackers | ½ cup |
| Graham (2½ inch) | 2 |
| Oyster | 20 (½ cup) |
| Saltines (2-inch square) | 5 |
| Soda (2½-inch square) | 3 |
| Round (1½-inch diameter) | 7 (omit 1 fat exchange) |
| Matzo (6-inch diameter) | 1 |
| Rye krisp | 4 |
| Rye thins | 10 (omit 1 fat exchange) |
| Triangle thins | 15 (omit 1 fat exchange) |
| Triscuit wafers | 5 |
| Vegetable thins | 10 |
| Wheat thins | 10 |
| Zweibach | 3 |
| Dutch pretzels | 1 |
| 3-ring pretzels | 5 |

| | |
|---|---|
| Thin pretzel sticks | 12 |
| Bacon thins | 15 (omit 2 fat exchanges) |
| French onion thins | 12 (omit 1 fat exchange) |
| Sesame thins | 10 (omit 2 fat exchanges) |
| Sociables | 12 (omit 1 fat exchange) |
| Vegetables—beans and peas, dried, cooked (lima, navy, split pea, cow peas, etc.) | ½ cup |
| Baked beans (no pork) | ¼ cup |
| Beans—fresh lima | ½ cup |
| Corn (6-inch ear) | ⅓ cup |
| Parsnips | ⅔ cup |
| Potatoes—white, baked, boiled | 1 (2-inch diameter) |
| mashed white | ½ cup |
| sweet or yams | ¼ cup |
| Sponge cake, plain | 1 (1½-inch cube) |
| Cupcake (no icing) | 1 (1¾-inch diameter) |
| Ice cream | ½ cup (omit 2 fat exchanges) |
| Jello | ½ cup (heaping) |
| Matzo meal | 2 tablespoons |
| Gingerbread | 1 small piece (omit 1 fat exchange) |
| Popcorn | 1 cup (omit 1 fat exchange) |
| Potato chips | 15 (omit 2 fat exchanges) |
| French fried potatoes—Bird's Eye | 12 (omit 1 fat exchange) |
| Tiny taters—Bird's Eye | 2.7 ounces (1/6 package) (omit 1 fat exchange) |
| Potato patty—Birds Eye | 1 (3 ounces) (omit 2 fat exchanges) |
| Onion rings | 2 ounces (omit 2 fat exchanges) |
| Dry bread crumbs | ¼ cup |
| Whip 'n Chill (made with all water) | ½ cup |
| Kool Pops—Bird's Eye | 2 pops |
| Donut | 1 (omit 1 fat exchange) |
| Ice cream cone | 1 |

| Fruit pop tart | ½ pop up |
| | (omit ½ fat exchange) |

## GENERAL MILLS' SNACKS

| Bugles, 15 pieces | ½ bread, 1 fat |
| Whistles, 14 pieces | ½ bread, ½ fat |
| Daisys, 24 pieces | ½ bread, ½ fat |
| Buttons, 40 pieces | ½ bread, ½ fat |
| Bows, 20 pieces | ½ bread, 1 fat |

## FRENCH'S POTATO PRODUCTS

| Scalloped potatoes (6 servings per package) 1 serving | 1½ bread |
| Potatoes Au Gratin (6 servings per package) 1 serving | 2 bread |
| Potato Pancakes (4 servings per package) 1 serving | 1½ bread |
| Instant Mashed Potatoes (4 servings per package) 1 serving | 2 bread |

## AUNT JEMIMA (made according to package directions)

| Pancake mix, three 4-inch pancakes (diameter) | 1½ bread |
| Buttermilk pancake mix, three 4-inch pancakes | 1¾ bread |
| Buckwheat pancake mix, three 4-inch pancakes | 1½ bread |
| Easy Pour pancake mix, three 4-inch pancakes | 2¼ bread |
| Corn bread easy mix, 1 slice 2¾ x 2⅝ x 1¼ -inch | 2¼ bread |

## FLAKO (made according to package directions)

| Pie crust, 1/6 of single 9-inch crust | ¾ bread |
| Cup cake mix, 1 cake 1½ x 2½-inch diameter | 1 bread |

37

Popover mix, 1 popover
    3½x3-inch diameter              1½ bread
Corn muffin mix, 1 muffin
    1⅜x2½-inch diameter          1½ bread

## CEREALS

### QUAKER OATS

| | |
|---|---|
| Life, ⅔ cup | 1 bread |
| Frosted Rice Puffs, 1 cup | 1 bread |
| Frosted Wheat Puffs, 1⅔ cup | 1 bread |
| Puffed Rice, 1½ cups | 1 bread |
| Puffed Wheat, 1⅔ cups | 1 bread |
| Quake, ¾ cup | 1 bread |
| Quisp, 1 cup | 1 bread |
| Shredded Wheat, 1 biscuit | 1½ bread |

### GENERAL MILLS

| | |
|---|---|
| Cheerios, 1 cup | 1 bread |
| Corn Bursts, ½ cup | 1 bread |
| Cocoa Puffs, ⅔ cup | 1 bread |
| Country Corn Flakes, 1 cup | 1 bread |
| Frosty O's, ⅔ cup | 1 bread |
| Jets, ½ cup | 1 bread |
| Kix, 1 cup | 1 bread |
| Lucky Charms, ¾ cup | 1 bread |
| Stax, 1 cup | 1 bread |
| Trix, ⅔ cup | 1 bread |
| Twinkles, ½ cup | 1 bread |
| Wheaties, ⅔ cup | 1 bread |
| Bran & Raisin Flavor Flakes, ⅔ cup | 1 bread |

# Absolutely Delicious Blueberry Muffins

| Ingredients | Measure | | Carbohydrates (gm.) | Protein (gm.) | Fat (gm.) |
|---|---|---|---|---|---|
| Bisquick | 2 | cups | 152 | 19 | 29 |
| Sour cream | 1 | cup | | | 40 |
| Egg | 1 | | | 7 | 5 |
| Fresh blueberries | 1 | cup | 15 | | |
| Artificial sweetener | = 6 | tablespoons sugar | | | |
| Lemon peel, grated | 2 | teaspoons | | | |
| | | | 167 | 26 | 74 |

Calories: 1 serving—119                         14    2    6

Preheat oven to 425 degrees. Combine Bisquick, ¼ cup artificial sweetener. Make well in center of mixture and add sour cream and egg, all at once. Beat with fork until well combined. Gently fold in blueberries. Put ¼ cup batter in each muffin cup. In small bowl combine lemon peel and 2 tablespoons artificial sweetener. Sprinkle over batter in each cup. Bake 20 to 25 minutes or until golden brown. Serve hot.

Servings: 12 muffins
Exchange per serving: 1 bread, 1 fat

# Corn Fritters

| Ingredients | Measure | Carbohydrates (gm.) | Protein (gm.) | Fat (gm.) |
|---|---|---|---|---|
| Frozen corn, cooked as directed | 2 cups | 90 | 12 | |
| Flour | 1 cup | 75.9 | 10.8 | .9 |
| Baking powder | 1 teaspoon | | | |
| Salt | ½ teaspoon | | | |
| Pepper | ¼ teaspoon | | | |
| Eggs, separated | 2 | | 14 | 10 |
| Milk | ½ cup | 6 | 4 | 5 |
| Oil for frying | | | | |
| | | 171.9 | 40.8 | 15.9 |
| Calories: 1 serving—54.6 | | 9.5 | 2.2 | .8 |

Sift flour, baking powder, salt and pepper. Beat egg whites until they form soft peaks. Beat egg yolks well; stir in corn and milk and flour mixture until blended; fold in egg whites.

Pour oil to depth of ½ inch and heat to medium. Drop rounded teaspoon of batter in oil and cook, turning once, 2 to 3 minutes, or until golden. Drain on paper towel.

Servings: 18
Exchange per serving: ¾ bread

RECIPE FOR

# Pineapple Fritters

| Ingredients | Measure | Carbohydrates (gm.) | Protein (gm.) | Fat (gm.) |
|---|---|---|---|---|
| Flour, sifted | 1 cup | 75.9 | 10.8 | .9 |
| Artificial sweetener | = 2 tablespoons sugar | | | |
| Baking powder | 2 teaspoons | | | |
| Salt | ¼ teaspoon | | | |
| Egg | 1 | | 7 | 5 |
| Milk | ⅔ cup | 8 | 6 | 6 |
| Margarine | 2 tablespoons | | | 30 |
| Pineapple, 10 slices, drained | 1 20-ounce can | 100 | | |
| | | 183.9 | 23.8 | 41.9 |
| Calories: 1 serving—116 | | 18 | 2 | 4 |

Sift flour, artificial sweetener, baking powder, and salt together. Mix egg, milk, and margarine together and stir into dry ingredients. Blend until smooth. Dip pineapple in batter, one at a time, and fry in hot fat (375 degrees) for 3 minutes, turning once. Drain on a paper towel and serve hot.

Servings: 10 fritters
Exchange per serving: 1 fruit, ½ bread, 1 fat

# Noodle Pudding

| Ingredients | Measure | Carbohydrates (gm.) | Protein (gm.) | Fat (gm.) |
|---|---|---|---|---|
| Wide noodles, cooked and drained | 10 ounces | 150 | 20 | |
| Eggs, beaten | 3 | | 21 | 15 |
| Artificial sweetener | = ¾ cup sugar | | | |
| Pineapple, crushed | 1 8-ounce can | 40 | | |
| Apples, peeled and grated | 5 | 50 | | |
| Maraschino cherries | 8 | 40 | | |
| Cinnamon | to taste | | | |
| Oil | 4 tablespoons | | | 60 |
| | | 280 | 41 | 75 |

Calories: 1 serving—108      17    2.5    4.5

Heat 1 tablespoon oil in pan. Combine remaining ingredients and pour into pan. Let set for 24 hours. Bake 1 hour at 350 degrees.

Servings: 16
Exchange per serving: 1 bread, 1 fat

RECIPE FOR

# Popovers

| Ingredients | Measure | Carbohydrates (gm.) | Protein (gm.) | Fat (gm.) |
|---|---|---|---|---|
| Eggs | 2 | | 14 | 10 |
| Milk, skim | 1 cup | 12 | 8 | |
| Flour | 1 cup | 75.9 | 10.8 | .9 |
| Salt | ¼ teaspoon | | | |
| Margarine, melted | 1 tablespoon | | | 15 |
| | | 87.9 | 32.8 | 25.9 |
| Calories: 1 serving—58.9 | | 7.3 | 2.7 | 2.1 |

Beat eggs and add milk as you continue to beat. Sift flour and salt together and add to egg and milk mixture as you continue to beat. Add melted margarine. Pour batter into 12 small popover cups. Bake at 425 degrees for 35 minutes.

Servings: 12
Exchange per serving: 1 vegetable B, ½ fat

# Quick Blender Popovers

| Ingredients | Measure | Carbohydrates (gm.) | Protein (gm.) | Fat (gm.) |
|---|---|---|---|---|
| Milk, skim | 1 cup | 12 | 8 | |
| Eggs | 2 | | 14 | 10 |
| Flour, sifted | 1 cup | 75.9 | 10.8 | .9 |
| Salt | ¼ teaspoon | | | |
| | | 87.9 | 32.8 | 10.9 |
| Calories: 1 serving—48.1 | | 7.3 | 2.7 | .9 |

Put all ingredients in blender. Cover and blend on high speed for 15 seconds. Pour into greased muffin pans and bake at 425 degrees for 40 minutes.

Servings: 12
Exchange per serving: 1 vegetable B

# Yorkshire Pudding

| Ingredients | Measure | Car-bohy-drates (gm.) | Pro-tein (gm.) | Fat (gm.) |
|---|---|---|---|---|
| Eggs | 2 | | 14 | 10 |
| Milk, skim | 1 cup | 12 | 8 | |
| Flour | 1 cup | 75.9 | 10.8 | .9 |
| Salt | ½ teaspoon | | | |
| Roast beef drippings | 2 tablespoons | | | |
| | | 87.9 | 32.8 | 10.9 |
| Calories: 1 serving—71.7 | | 10.9 | 4.1 | 1.3 |

As soon as roast beef has been removed from the oven, increase oven temperature to 425 degrees. In a medium bowl beat eggs, milk, flour, and salt to make a smooth batter. Pour drippings into a 10-inch pie plate (or six individual custard cups); tilt to coat bottom and side of pie plate. Pour in batter. Bake 25 minutes or until the pudding is deep golden brown. Serve immediately with the roast beef.

Servings: 8
Exchange per serving: ½ milk, ½ fruit or 1 fruit, ½ meat

# Muffins

| Ingredients | Measure | Carbohydrates (gm.) | Protein (gm.) | Fat (gm.) |
|---|---|---|---|---|
| Flour | 1½ cups | 113.8 | 16.2 | 1.3 |
| Double-acting baking powder | 3 teaspoons | | | |
| Salt | ½ teaspoon | | | |
| Egg, slightly beaten | 1 | | 7 | 5 |
| Milk, skim | ¾ cup | 9 | 6 | |
| Vegetable oil | 2 tablespoons | | | 30 |
| Artificial sweetener | = 8 teaspoon sugar | | | |
| | | 122.8 | 29.2 | 36.3 |
| Calories: 1 serving—116.1 | | 15.2 | 3.6 | 4.5 |

Sift flour, baking powder, and salt together. Combine egg, milk, oil, and artificial sweetener. Add liquid mixture to dry ingredients, mixing until all dry particles are moistened. Fill well greased muffin cups two-thirds full. Bake at 400 degrees for 25 minutes.

Servings: 8
Exchange per serving: 1 bread, 1 fat

# Apple Muffins

| Ingredients | Measure | Car-bohy-drates (gm.) | Pro-tein (gm.) | Fat (gm.) |
|---|---|---|---|---|
| Flour | 1⅔ cups | 128.9 | 18.2 | 1.5 |
| Artificial sweetener | = 16 teaspoons sugar | | | |
| Baking powder | 2½ teaspoons | | | |
| Salt | ½ teaspoon | | | |
| Cinnamon | 1 teaspoon | | | |
| Nutmeg | ¼ teaspoon | | | |
| Egg, lightly beaten | 1 | | 7 | 5 |
| Milk | ⅔ cup | 8 | 6 | 6 |
| Margarine, melted | ¼ cup | | | 60 |
| Apples, minced | 1 cup | 20 | | |
| | | 156.9 | 31.2 | 72.5 |

Calories: 1 serving—116.4

| | | 13 | 2.6 | 6 |
|---|---|---|---|---|

Sift flour, artificial sweetener, baking powder, salt, and spices into mixing bowl. Combine egg, milk, and margarine; add to dry ingredients. Blend until flour is moistened. Do not overmix or batter will be lumpy. Fold in apples. Pour batter into greased muffin cups filling until two-thirds full. Bake at 400 degrees for 25 minutes.

Servings: 12
Exchange per serving: 1 bread, 1 fat

# Orange Marmalade Nut Bread

| Ingredients | Measure | Carbohydrates (gm.) | Protein (gm.) | Fat (gm.) |
|---|---|---|---|---|
| Flour | 2 cups | 151.8 | 21.6 | 1.8 |
| Baking powder | 1½ teaspoon | | | |
| Baking soda | ½ teaspoon | | | |
| Salt | ¼ teaspoon | | | |
| Milk, skim | ⅓ cup | 4 | 2.6 | |
| Egg | 1 | | 7 | 5 |
| Margarine, melted | 2 tablespoons | | | 30 |
| Artificial sweetener | = 8 tablespoons sugar | | | |
| Dietetic orange marmalade | ½ cup | | | |
| Walnuts, chopped | ¼ cup | | | 20 |
| | | 155.8 | 31.2 | 56.8 |
| Calories: 1 serving—104.3 | | 12.9 | 2.6 | 4.7 |

Combine flour, baking powder, baking soda, and salt in a mixing bowl. Combine milk, egg, margarine, and artificial sweetener; add to flour mixture. Stir only until all flour is moistened. Fold in marmalade and chopped nuts, mixing as little as possible. Spoon batter into lightly greased loaf pan. Bake at 350 degrees for 1 hour. Cool before slicing.

Servings: 12
Exchange per serving: 1 bread, 1 fat

# Banana Nut Bread

| Ingredients | Measure | Carbohydrates (gm.) | Protein (gm.) | Fat (gm.) |
|---|---|---|---|---|
| Ripe bananas, mashed | 3 | 60 | | |
| Artificial sweetener, granulated | = 24 teaspoons sugar | | | |
| Eggs, well beaten | 2 | | 14 | 10 |
| Flour | 1¾ cups | 132.7 | 18.9 | 1.5 |
| Baking powder | 3 teaspoons | | | |
| Salt | ¼ teaspoon | | | |
| Walnuts, chopped | ¼ cup | | | 20 |
| | | 192.7 | 32.9 | 31.5 |
| Calories: 1 serving—98.2 | | 16 | 2.7 | 2.6 |

Sprinkle artificial sweetener over bananas and mix well; blend in eggs. Sift together flour, baking powder, and salt; add walnuts; blend thoroughly into banana mixture but do not overmix. Pour into loaf pan. Bake at 325 degrees for 55 minutes.

Servings: 12
Exchange per serving: 1 bread, ½ fat

# Stuffed Baked Potatoes

| Ingredients | Measure | Carbohydrates (gm.) | Protein (gm.) | Fat (gm.) |
|---|---|---|---|---|
| Baking potatoes | 4 | 60 | 8 | |
| Onion, minced | ¼ cup | 3.5 | 1 | |
| Salt | 1 teaspoon | | | |
| Pepper | ⅛ teaspoon | | | |
| Margarine | 1 tablespoon | | | 15 |
| Egg | 1 | | 7 | 5 |
| Sour cream | 4 tablespoons | | | 10 |
| | | 63.5 | 16 | 30 |

Calories: 1 serving—146.7    15.8   4   7.5

Bake potatoes at 400 degrees for 1 hour. Remove from oven and cut in half lengthwise. Remove pulp, reserving skins. Place pulp in mixing bowl. Add onion, salt, pepper, margarine, and egg. Beat well, until fluffy. Refill potato skins and arrange in a shallow baking dish with cut sides up. Spoon sour cream over each half. Bake 10 minutes until tops are lightly browned.

Servings: 4
Exchange per serving: 1 bread, 1½ fat

# Oven Browned Potato Sticks

| Ingredients | Measure | Car-bohy-drates (gm.) | Pro-tein (gm.) | Fat (gm.) |
|---|---|---|---|---|
| Large potatoes, sliced into sticks | 8 | 120 | 16 | |
| Salad oil | ½ cup | | | 120 |
| Salt | 1 teaspoon | | | |
| | | 120 | 16 | 120 |
| Calories: 1 serving—203 | | 15 | 2 | 15 |

Place salad oil in a large shallow baking pan; roll potato sticks in oil to coat well, then arrange in a single layer in same pan; sprinkle with salt. Bake at 400 degrees for 1 hour, or until tender and crusty-golden.

Servings: 8
Exchange per serving: 1 bread, 3 fat

# Potato Cake

| Ingredients | Measure | Car- bohy- drates (gm.) | Pro- tein (gm.) | Fat (gm.) |
|---|---|---|---|---|
| Medium potatoes, peeled | 6 | 90 | 12 | |
| Margarine | 4 tablespoons | | | 60 |
| Salt | as desired | | | |
| Pepper | as desired | | | |
| | | 90 | 12 | 60 |
| Calories: 1 serving—158 | | 15 | 2 | 10 |

Slice potatoes thinly and evenly. Butter 1½-quart baking dish. Arrange layer of potatoes over bottom and sides. Dot with margarine. Sprinkle with salt and pepper. Repeat until dish is full. Cover. Bake at 400 degrees for 1 hour. Carefully turn out on warm platter.

Servings: 6
Exchange per serving: 1 bread, 2 fat

# Escalloped Potatoes

| Ingredients | Measure | Carbohydrates (gm.) | Protein (gm.) | Fat (gm.) |
|---|---|---|---|---|
| Potato, peeled | 1 small | 15 | 2 | |
| Salt | as desired | | | |
| Pepper | as desired | | | |
| Onion, chopped | ½ teaspoon | | | |
| Milk, skim | ½ cup | 6 | 4 | |
| Margarine | 1 teaspoon | | | 5 |
| Calories: 1 serving—153 | | 21 | 6 | 5 |

Slice potato and place half the slices in bottom of individual casserole. Sprinkle lightly with salt, pepper, and chopped onion. Cover with remaining potato slices; sprinkle with salt and pepper and add milk. Dot top with margarine. Bake in moderate oven (350 degrees) about 45 minutes.

Servings: 1
Exchange per serving: 1 bread, ½ milk

# Quick Scalloped Potatoes

| Ingredients | Measure | | Carbohy-drates (gm.) | Pro-tein (gm.) | Fat (gm.) |
|---|---|---|---|---|---|
| Cheddar cheese soup | 1 | 10½-ounce can | 24.9 | 14.4 | 29.7 |
| Milk, skim | ½ | cup | 6 | 4 | |
| Potatoes, thinly sliced | 4 | cups | 60 | 8 | |
| Onion, thinly sliced | 1 | | 7 | 2 | |
| Margarine | 1 | tablespoon | | | 15 |
| Paprika | | as desired | | | |
| | | | 97.9 | 28.4 | 44.7 |
| Calories: 1 serving—150.6 | | | 16.3 | 4.7 | 7.4 |

Stir soup until smooth; gradually add milk. In buttered casserole arrange alternate layers of potato, onion, and the cheese sauce. Dot top with margarine. Sprinkle with paprika. Bake, covered, at 375 degrees for 1 hour. Uncover, bake 15 minutes more.

Servings: 6
Exchange per serving: 1 bread, 1½ fat

# Crisp Baked Potato Halves

| Ingredients | Measure | | Carbohydrates (gm.) | Protein (gm.) | Fat (gm.) |
|---|---|---|---|---|---|
| Baking potatoes | 4 | medium | 60 | 8 | |
| Margarine | 4 | tablespoons | | | 60 |
| Salt | | as desired | | | |
| Pepper | | as desired | | | |
| | | | 60 | 8 | 60 |
| Calories: 1 serving—203 | | | 15 | 2 | 15 |

Scrub potatoes and cut in half lengthwise. Score cut side of each half with a fork; brush with margarine and sprinkle with salt and pepper. Place potatoes on a cookie sheet, cut sides up, and bake at 400 degrees for 40 minutes, until fork tender.

Servings: 4
Exchange per serving: 1 bread, 3 fat

# Potato Salad

| Ingredients | Measure | Car-bohy-drates (gm.) | Pro-tein (gm.) | Fat (gm.) |
|---|---|---|---|---|
| Potatoes, cooked and finely diced | 6 cups (6) | 90 | 12 | |
| Onion, grated | 1 | 7 | 2 | |
| Chopped dill pickle | 3 tablespoons | | | |
| Mayonnaise | ½ cup | | | 120 |
| Prepared mustard | 1½ teaspoons | | | |
| Salt | ½ teaspoon | | | |
| Pepper | ⅛ teaspoon | | | |
| | | 97 | 14 | 120 |
| Calories: 1 serving—253.6 | | 16.1 | 2.3 | 20 |

Combine all ingredients and refrigerate. You can use this recipe for macaroni salad by substituting 3 cups cooked macaroni for the potatoes.

Servings: 6
Exchange per serving: 1 bread, 4 fat

# Mushroom Potato Pie

| Ingredients | Measure | Carbohydrates (gm.) | Protein (gm.) | Fat (gm.) |
|---|---|---|---|---|
| Potatoes, mashed | 3 cups | 90 | 12 | |
| Mushrooms, sliced | 1½ cups | | | |
| Onion, minced | ¼ cup | 3.5 | 1 | |
| Margarine | 2 tablespoons | | | 30 |
| Lemon juice | 1 teaspoon | | | |
| Salt | as desired | | | |
| Pepper | ⅛ teaspoon | | | |
| Sour cream | ½ cup | | | 20 |
| | | 93.5 | 13 | 50 |

Calories: 1 serving→145.1    15.5    2.1    8.3

Place half the mashed potatoes in a layer in a buttered 9-inch pie pan. Sauté mushrooms and onion in hot margarine. Stir in lemon juice, salt, and pepper. Top potatoes with mushrooms and sour cream. Cover with remaining potatoes. Bake at 350 degrees about 35 minutes.

Servings: 6
Exchange per serving: 1 bread, 1½ fat

# Potato and Onion in Foil

| Ingredients | Measure | Carbohydrates (gm.) | Protein (gm.) | Fat (gm.) |
|---|---|---|---|---|
| Baking potato | 1 medium | 15 | 2 | |
| Onion, thinly sliced | 1 medium | 7 | 2 | |
| Margarine | 2 teaspoons | | | 10 |
| Salt | ½ teaspoon | | | |
| Paprika | as desired | | | |
| Calories: 1 serving—194 | | 22 | 4 | 10 |

Place potato, cut into ¼-inch slices, on piece of aluminum foil. Insert an onion slice between each 2 potato slices. Spread potato with margarine, salt, and paprika. Bring foil together and fold over to seal. Place on baking sheet. Bake at 425 degrees for 45 minutes, or until tender.

Servings: 1
Exchange per serving: 1 bread, 1 vegetable B, 2 fat

# Bread Stuffing

| Ingredients | Measure | Car-bohy-drates (gm.) | Pro-tein (gm.) | Fat (gm.) |
|---|---|---|---|---|
| Bread | 1 slice | 15 | 2 | |
| Onion, chopped | ½ teaspoon | | | |
| Salt | pinch | | | |
| Pepper | few grains | | | |
| Poultry seasoning | ⅛ teaspoon | | | |
| Margarine, melted | 1 teaspoon | | | 5 |
| Water | to moisten | | | |
| Calories: 1 serving—113 | | 15 | 2 | 5 |

Cut bread into cubes. Add onion, seasonings, and margarine; mix well. Add water to moisten.

Servings: 1
Exchange per serving: 1 bread, 1 fat

# CHAPTER VI

# Meat

## MEAT

*1 meat exchange consists of*:

| | | |
|---|---|---|
| Protein | 7 gm. | |
| Fat | 5 gm. | |
| Calories | 73 | |

| | |
|---|---|
| Meat and poultry (medium fat) (beef, lamb, pork, liver, chicken, etc.) | 1 ounce |
| Cold cuts (4½-inch square, ⅛-inch thick) | 1 slice |
| Frankfurter | 1 (8-9 per pound) |
| Fish | |
| (cod, mackerel, etc., | 1 ounce |
| salmon, tuna, crab, | ¼ cup |
| oysters, shrimp, clams, | 5 small |
| sardines) | 3 medium |
| Cheese | |
| (Cheddar, American, Swiss, | 1 ounce |
| cottage) | ¼ cup |
| Eggs | 1 |
| Peanut butter (limit use to 2 tablespoons per day) | 2 tablespoons |
| Fish sticks (Mrs. Paul's) | 1½ (omit ½ bread exchange) |
| Fish patties (Mrs. Paul's) | 1 (omit ½ bread exchange) |

1 egg

| | | | |
|---|---|---|---|
| whole | .3 Carbohydrate | 6.1 Protein | 5.5 Fat |
| white | .2 Carbohydrate | 3.3 Protein | 0 Fat |
| yolk | .1 Carbohydrate | 2.8 Protein | 5.4 Fat |

| | |
|---|---|
| Caviar | 2 rounded teaspoons |
| Sardines, in oil | 7 medium (omit 1 fat exchange) |

| | |
|---|---|
| Sardines, in tomato sauce | ½ large |
| Shrimp | 5 |
| Lobster | ¼ cup |
| Clams | 5 |

## BROILING:

Meat broiled can be calculated as 1 meat exchange per ounce of cooked meat.

### Suitable cuts for broiling

| *Beef* | *Pork* |
|---|---|
| Club steak | Bacon |
| Top quality chuck steak | Ham |
| Patties | Loin chops |
| Porterhouse steak | Rib chops |
| Tenderloin | Shoulder chops |
| Top quality top round | *Veal* |
| T-bone steak | Loin chops |
| Rib steak | |
| Sirloin steak | |
| *Lamb* | |
| Loin chops | |
| Rib chops | |
| Shoulder chops | |
| Patties | |
| Steak | |

## PAN BROILING:

Meat pan broiled (in Teflon pans to eliminate the use of fat) can be calculated as 1 meat exchange per ounce of cooked meat.

### Suitable cuts for pan broiling

| | |
|---|---|
| Bacon | Lamb chops |
| Beef or lamb patties | Sausage |
| Cubed steak | Steaks, less than 1-inch thick |
| Ham | |

*ROASTING*:

Meat roasted can be calculated as 1 meat exchange per ounce of cooked meat.

### Suitable cuts for roasting

*Beef*—300°
Choice quality chuck ribs
Rolled ribs
Rump
Standing ribs
Tenderloin
Choice quality top round
*Lamb* 300°
Crown roast
Leg
Loin
Ribs
Shoulder

*Pork* 350°
Boston butt
Crown roast
Fresh or smoked ham
Loin
Picnic shoulder
*Veal* 300°
Leg
Loin
Shoulder

Roast in slow oven, on rack, without adding water or other liquid. Roast 20 to 30 minutes per pound for beef; 25 to 40 minutes per pound for veal; 25 to 45 minutes per pound for pork; 30 to 40 minutes per pound for lamb.

### Internal temperatures of roasts when done

| Cut | Rare | Medium | Well done |
|-----|------|--------|-----------|
| Beef | 140° | 160° | 170° |
| Lamb | | 175° | 180° |
| Pork | | | 185° |
| Veal | | | 170° |
| Ham | | | 170° |

# Liver and Onion

| Ingredients | Measure | Carbohydrates (gm.) | Protein (gm.) | Fat (gm.) |
|---|---|---|---|---|
| Margarine | 6 tablespoons | | | 90 |
| Onion, frozen, chopped | 1½ cups | 21 | 6 | |
| Flour | ¼ cup | 19 | 2.7 | .2 |
| Salt | 2 teaspoons | | | |
| Paprika | 2 teaspoons | | | |
| Beef liver, sliced | 2 pounds | | 168 | 120 |
| | | 40 | 176.7 | 210.2 |

Calories: 1 serving—453     6.4   28   35

Combine 4 tablespoons margarine and onions in frying pan; heat slowly until margarine melts; cover pan and cook slowly 5 minutes. Uncover and cook, stirring several times, 10 minutes or until golden. Mix flour, salt, and paprika in pie plate and coat liver pieces. Sauté in remaining margarine in frying pan 4 minutes on each side, or until done as you like it. Serve on serving platter and surround with onions.

Servings: 6
Exchange per serving: 4 meat, ½ bread, 3 fat

# Baked Tongue

| Ingredients | Measure | Carbohydrates (gm.) | Protein (gm.) | Fat (gm.) |
|---|---|---|---|---|
| Tongue, pickled or smoked | | | | |
| Water | ½ cup | | | |

Place tongue in casserole; add water; cover and bake at 350 degrees for 50 minutes per pound.

Exchange per serving: 1 meat exchange per ounce in serving

# Danish Salad Mold

| Ingredients | Measure | Carbohydrates (gm.) | Protein (gm.) | Fat (gm.) |
|---|---|---|---|---|
| Potatoes, cooked and finely diced | 6 cups (6) | 90 | 12 | |
| Onion, grated | 1 | 7 | 2 | |
| Chopped dill pickle | 3 tablespoons | | | |
| Mayonnaise | ½ cup | | | 120 |
| Prepared mustard | 1½ teaspoon | | | |
| Salt | ½ teaspoon | | | |
| Pepper | ⅛ teaspoon | | | |
| Beef tongue, cooked | 12 1-ounce slices | | 84 | 35 |
| Lettuce | | | | |
| | | 97 | 98 | 155 |
| Calories: 1 serving—361.8 | | 16.1 | 16.3 | 25.8 |

Combine potatoes, onion, pickle, mayonnaise, and seasonings; mix well. Line lightly oiled 6-cup mixing bowl with tongue slices, slightly overlapping, with rounded ends toward bottom of bowl; fill with potato salad mixture, pressing down lightly all over to fill bowl. Chill 1 hour. When ready to serve loosen meat around edge of bowl; turn bowl upside down on serving plate and lift off. Garnish with lettuce.

Servings: 6

Exchange per serving: 2 meat, 1 bread, 3 fat

# Combination Salad

| Ingredients | Measure | Car-bohy-drates (gm.) | Pro-tein (gm.) | Fat (gm.) |
|---|---|---|---|---|
| American cheese, in strips | 1 ounce | | 7 | 5 |
| Cold cuts, in strips | 2 ounces | | 14 | 10 |
| Egg, hard boiled | 1 | | 7 | 5 |
| Lettuce, shredded | ¼ Small head | | | |
| Onion, sliced | 1 small | | | |
| Tomato, quartered | 1 | | | |
| Raw cauliflowerets, asparagus spears, peas, etc., cooked | as desired | | | |
| Vinegar | 2 tablespoons | | | |
| Salad oil | 2 teaspoons | | | 10 |
| Calories: 1 serving—292 | | | 28 | 30 |

Combine first 7 ingredients; season as desired. Pour vinegar over; pour oil over and toss to coat well.

Servings: 1
Exchange per serving: 4 meat, ½ bread

# Flank Steak

| Ingredients | Measure | Carbohydrates (gm.) | Protein (gm.) | Fat (gm.) |
|---|---|---|---|---|
| Flank steak | 1 pound | | 84 | 60 |
| Vegetable oil | 1 cup | | | |
| Vinegar | ½ cup | | | |
| Salt | 1 teaspoon | | | |
| Pepper | ¼ teaspoon | | | |
| Dry mustard | 2 teaspoons | | | |
| Worcestershire sauce | 2 teaspoons | | | |
| Cayenne | dash | | | |
| Tabasco sauce | few drops | | | |

Calrories: 1 serving—219

Place steak in pan. Combine remaining ingredients and pour over steak. Let stand at least 3 hours. Remove from marinade and broil 5 minutes on each side 2 inches from fire. Carve diagonally across grain into thin slices. (Discard marinade.)

Servings: 4
Exchange per serving: 3 meat

# Chopped Chicken Livers

| Ingredients | Measure | | Carbohydrates (gm.) | Protein (gm.) | Fat (gm.) |
|---|---|---|---|---|---|
| Oil | 2 | tablespoons | | | 30 |
| Onions, sliced | 2 | small | 14 | 4 | |
| Chicken livers | ½ | pound | | 42 | 30 |
| Water | 2 | tablespoons | | | |
| Eggs, hard cooked, chopped | 2 | | | 14 | 10 |
| Salt | ½ | teaspoon | | | |
| Pepper | | few grains | | | |
| Chicken broth | 3 | tablespoons | | | |
| | | | 14 | 60 | 70 |
| Calories: 1 2-ounce serving—185.2 | | | 28 | 12 | 14 |

Heat oil in skillet; add onion and cook until tender, stirring occasionally. Add livers and cook until lightly browned. Add water; cover and cook slowly 10 minutes. Cool and chop livers finely. Mix livers, egg, salt, and pepper. Stir in broth to moisten.

Servings: 5
Exchange per serving: 1½ meat, 1½ fat

# CHAPTER VII

# Beef

# Beef Stew With Dumplings

| Ingredients | Measure | | Car-bohy-drates (gm.) | Pro-tein (gm.) | Fat (gm.) |
|---|---|---|---|---|---|
| Boneless beef chuck, cut into 1-inch cubes | 1 | pound | | 84 | 60 |
| Hot water | 2 | cups | | | |
| Lemon juice | ½ | teaspoon | | | |
| Worcestershire sauce | ½ | teaspoon | | | |
| Garlic, minced | ½ | clove | | | |
| Onion, sliced | ½ | | | | |
| Bay leaf, crumbled | 1 | small | | | |
| Salt | 1 | teaspoon | | | |
| Pepper | ¼ | teaspoon | | | |
| Artificial sweetener = | ½ | teaspoon sugar | | | |
| Carrots, halved | 3 | | 21 | 6 | |
| Onions | 4 | small | 14 | 4 | |
| Potatoes, quartered | 2 | | 30 | 4 | |
| Dumplings (recipe below) | | | 80.5 | 12.5 | 14.5 |
| | | | 145.5 | 110.5 | 74.5 |
| Calories: 1 serving—423 | | | 36.3 | 27.6 | 18.6 |

Brown meat thoroughly on all sides (about 30 minutes) in heavy pan. Add all ingredients except vegetables. Cover tightly. Cook 2 hours. Add vegetables, cook 10 minutes. Add dumplings; finish cooking with dumplings.

Servings: 4
Exchange per serving: 2 bread, 3 meat, 1 vegetable B, 1 fat

# Dumplings

| Ingredients | Measure | Carbohydrates (gm.) | Protein (gm.) | Fat (gm.) |
|---|---|---|---|---|
| Bisquick | 1 cup | 76 | 9.5 | 14.5 |
| Milk, skim | 6 tablespoons | 4.5 | 3 | |
| | | 80.5 | 12.5 | 14.5 |
| Calories: 1 serving—125.2 | | 20.1 | 3.1 | 3.6 |

Mix milk with bisquick. Spoon batter lightly onto bubbling stew. Cook 10 lings on warm plates.

Servings: 4
minutes uncovered and 10 minutes covered. Remove. Top stew with dump-
Exchange per serving: 1½ bread, ½ fat

# Barbecued Chuck Roast

| Ingredients | Measure | Car-bohy-drates (gm.) | Pro-tein (gm.) | Fat (gm.) |
|---|---|---|---|---|
| Chuck roast, boneless | 2 pounds, 2-inches thick | | 168 | 120 |
| Monosodium glutamate | 1 teaspoon | | | |
| Wine vinegar | ⅓ cup | | | |
| Catsup | ¼ cup | 19.6 | 1.6 | |
| Salad oil | 2 tablespoons | | | 30 |
| Soy sauce | 2 tablespoons | | | |
| Worcestershire sauce | 1 tablespoon | | | |
| Garlic salt | 1 teaspoon | | | |
| Prepared mustard | 1 teaspoon | | | |
| Pepper | ¼ teaspoon | | | |
| | | 19.6 | 169.6 | 150 |
| Calories: 1 serving—256.4 | | 2.4 | 21.2 | 18 |

Wipe meat, sprinkle with monosodium glutamate, and place in shallow baking dish. Combine all remaining ingredients; mix well; pour over meat and refrigerate, covered, 2 to 3 hours, turning meat several times. Take meat out of marinade, sprinkle with monosodium glutamate, and broil 6 inches from heat for 50 minutes, turning every 10 minutes and brushing with marinade.

Servings: 8
Exchange per serving: 3 meat, ½ fat

# Brisket Dinner

| Ingredients | Measure | Carbohydrates (gm.) | Protein (gm.) | Fat (gm.) |
|---|---|---|---|---|
| Beef brisket, boneless | 2 pounds | | 168 | 120 |
| Water | 1 cup | | | |
| Beef bouillon cubes | 2 | | | |
| Garlic, minced | 1 clove | | | |
| Bay leaf | 1 | | | |
| Onion, peeled | 1 | | | |
| Cloves, whole | 8 | | | |
| Onions, peeled | 4 | 28 | 8 | |
| Carrots, in 2-inch cubes | 6 | 28 | 8 | |
| Salt | 2 teaspoons | | | |
| Pepper | ¼ teaspoon | | | |
| Mushrooms, fresh | 6 large | | | |
| Flour | 3 tablespoons | 33.3 | 4.5 | |
| | | 89.3 | 188.5 | 120 |

Calories: 1 serving—273.8      11.1   23.6   15

Brown beef; stir in water, bouillon cubes, garlic, and bay leaf. Stud onion with cloves; drop into pan; cover. Simmer 1½ hours, turning meat once. Place onions and carrots in liquid around meat, sprinkle with salt and pepper, and cover again. Simmer 45 minutes. Add mushrooms and simmer 15 minutes. Remove meat to heated platter, place vegetables around edge, discarding bay leaf and onion with cloves; keep hot while making gravy.

Pour liquid into 4-cup measure; let stand about a minute. Skim off fat and measure 3 tablespoons back into pan. Add water, if needed, to make 3 cups. Blend flour into fat in pan; cook, stirring constantly, just until bubbly. Stir in the 3 cups liquid; continue cooking, stirring constantly, until gravy thickens and boils one minute. Serve slices of meat with gravy.

Servings: 8
Exchange per serving: 3 meat, 1 fruit

# Lipton Pot Roast in Onion Sauce

| Ingredients | Measure | Carbohydrates (gm.) | Protein (gm.) | Fat (gm.) |
|---|---|---|---|---|
| Boneless pot roast of beef | 3 to 4 pounds | | 252 | 180 |
| Water | 2 cups | | | |
| Lipton onion soup mix | 1 envelope | 30 | 4 | |

Brown meat well. Add water and soup mix. Simmer, covered, 3 hours, or until meat is tender, turning occasionally.

Exchange per serving: 1 meat exchange per ounce serving

# Man-Style Meat and Potatoes

| Ingredients | Measure | Car-bohy-drates (gm.) | Pro-tein (gm.) | Fat (gm.) |
|---|---|---|---|---|
| Beef, cooked, cut into strips | 1½ cups | | 84 | 60 |
| Onion, thinly sliced | 1 | 7 | 2 | |
| Margarine | 2 tablespoons | | | 30 |
| Cream of celery soup | 1 10½-ounce can | 19.2 | 4.2 | 11.7 |
| Milk | ⅓ cup | 4 | 2.6 | 3.3 |
| Cheddar cheese, shredded | 1 cup | | 28 | 20 |
| Pepper | dash | | | |
| Potatoes, cooked and sliced | 3 cups | 90 | 12 | |
| Paprika | dash | | | |
| | | 120.2 | 132.8 | 125 |
| Calories: 1 serving—534 | | 30 | 33.8 | 31 |

In sauce pan, brown beef and cook onion in margarine until onion is tender. Blend in soup, milk, ¾ cup cheese, and pepper. In a 1½-quart casserole arrange alternating layers of potatoes, meat, onion, and sauce. Sprinkle with remaining cheese and paprika. Bake uncovered at 375 degrees for 30 minutes.

Servings: 4
Exchange per serving: 2 bread, 4 meat, 2 fat

# Steak-Potato Casserole

| Ingredients | Measure | Car-bohy-drates (gm.) | Pro-tein (gm.) | Fat (gm.) |
|---|---|---|---|---|
| Round steak | 1 pound | | 84 | 60 |
| Flour | 2 tablespoons | 22.4 | 3 | |
| Margarine | 3 tablespoons | | | 45 |
| Potatoes, peeled and sliced | 4 | 60 | 8 | |
| Onion, chopped | | 1 | | |
| Parsley, chopped | few sprigs | | | |
| Salt | ½ teaspoon | | | |
| Pepper | ⅛ teaspoon | | | |
| Tomato sauce | 16 ounces | 56 | 16 | |
| | | 138.4 | 111 | 105 |
| Calories: 1 serving—482 | | 34.6 | 28 | 26 |

Cut meat into 4 serving pieces and dredge in flour. Brown in margarine on both sides in dutch oven. Add potatoes and next four ingredients. Pour tomato sauce over top. Cover and bake in moderate oven (350 degrees) about 1½ hours.

Servings: 4
Exchange per serving: 3 meat, 2½ bread, 2 fat

# Spanish Rice—Using Leftover Beef

| Ingredients | Measure | Car- bohy- drates (gm.) | Pro- tein (gm.) | Fat (gm.) |
|---|---|---|---|---|
| Green pepper, chopped | ½ cup | | | |
| Onion, chopped | ½ cup | 7 | 2 | |
| Rice, cooked | 1½ cups | 45 | 6 | |
| Oil | ¼ cup | | | 60 |
| Beef broth | 1 cup | | | |
| Tomato sauce | 16 ounces | 56 | 16 | |
| Salt | ½ teaspoon | | | |
| Pepper | ⅛ teaspoon | | | |
| Beef, cooked and diced | 1½ cups | | 84 | 60 |
| | | 108 | 108 | 120 |
| Calories: 1 serving—486 | | 27 | 27 | 30 |

Saute green pepper, onion and rice in oil, stirring until lightly brown. Add broth, tomato sauce, salt, pepper and beef. Bring to boil, reduce heat, and simmer uncovered 5 minutes.

Servings: 4
Exchange per serving: 3 meat, 2 bread, 3 fat

# CHAPTER VIII

# Lamb and Veal

# Shoulder Lamb Chops, Shaslik Style

| Ingredients | Measure | Carbohydrates (gm.) | Protein (gm.) | Fat (gm.) |
|---|---|---|---|---|
| Shoulder lamb chops | 6 5-ounce chops, excluding bone | | 168 | 120 |
| Vegetable oil | ½ cup | | | |
| Red wine vinegar | 2 tablespoons | | | |
| Lemon juice | 2 tablespoons | | | |
| Garlic salt | 1 teaspoon | | | |
| Pepper | ¼ teaspoon | | | |
| Oregano | ½ teaspoon | | | |
| Bay leaf, crumpled | ½ | | | |

Calories: 1 serving—292

Place chops in shallow pan. Mix remaining ingredients, pour over chops, cover. Marinate at least 24 hours, turning occasionally. Remove chops from marinade and broil 3 inches from fire about 12 minutes. (Discard marinade.)

Servings: 6
Exchange per serving: 4 meat

# Glazed Lamb Chops with Onions

| Ingredients | Measure | Carbohydrates (gm.) | Protein (gm.) | Fat (gm.) |
|---|---|---|---|---|
| Shoulder lamb chops | 8 5-ounce chops excluding bone | | 224 | 160 |
| Small white onions, drained | 1 16-ounce can | 28 | 8 | |
| Frozen orange juice concentrate | 1 6-ounce can | 60 | | |
| Salt | as desired | | | |
| Pepper | as desired | | | |
| | | 88 | 232 | 160 |
| Calories: 1 serving—340 | | 11 | 29 | 20 |

Season chops with salt and pepper and lightly brown on both sides in skillet. Arrange chops and onions in shallow roasting pan. Heat orange juice concentrate with pan drippings; pour over chops. Cover. Bake at 350 degrees for 30 minutes. Uncover; bake 15 minutes more, or until tender, basting frequently.

Servings: 8
Exchange per serving: 4 meat, 1 fruit

# Shish Kabob

| Ingredients | Measure | Carbohydrates (gm.) | Protein (gm.) | Fat (gm.) |
|---|---|---|---|---|
| Leg of lamb, cut into 1½-inch cubes | 4 ounces (raw) | | 21 | 15 |
| Onion, quartered | 1 | 7 | 2 | |
| Green pepper | 1 | | | |
| Cherry tomatoes | 4 | | | |
| Mushrooms | 6 | | | |
| Calories: 1 serving—255 | | 7 | 23 | 15 |

Alternate lamb cubes and vegetables on skewer. Brush cubes with barbecue sauce. Broil 4 inches from heat for 25 minutes, turning frequently.

Servings: 1
Exchange per serving: 3 meat, 1 vegetable **B**

# Veal Parmigiana

| Ingredients | Measure | Carbohydrates (gm.) | Protein (gm.) | Fat (gm.) |
|---|---|---|---|---|
| Veal steak, very thin | 1 pound | | 84 | 60 |
| Onion, minced | 1 | 7 | 2 | |
| Olive oil | 3 tablespoons | | | 45 |
| Tomatoes | 1 19-ounce can | | | |
| Garlic salt | 1¼ teaspoons | | | |
| Pepper | ¼ teaspoon | | | |
| Tomato sauce | 1 8-ounce can | 28 | 8 | |
| Oregano | dash | | | |
| Dry bread crumbs | ¼ cup | 15 | 2 | |
| Parmesan cheese, grated | 2 ounces | | 14 | 10 |
| Egg, beaten | 1 | | 7 | 5 |
| Mozzarella cheese | ½ Pound | | 56 | 40 |
| | | 50 | 173 | 160 |
| Calories: 1 serving—581.6 | | 12.2 | 43.2 | 40 |

Cut veal in serving-size pieces. Cook onion in 1 tablespoon olive oil 5 minutes. Add tomatoes, broken with fork; add garlic salt and pepper. Simmer, uncovered, 10 minutes. Add tomato sauce and oregano. Simmer 20 minutes longer. Mix bread crumbs and ¼ cup grated cheese. Dip veal in egg, then in crumbs. Brown in 2 tablespoons oil in skillet. Put in shallow baking dish. Pour about ⅔ sauce over veal; top with mozzarella, then rest of sauce. Sprinkle with grated cheese. Bake at 375 degrees for 30 minutes.

Servings: 4
Exchange per serving: 1 whole milk, 5 meat, 1 fat

# CHAPTER IX

# Ground Meat

# Meat Loaf Cake

| Ingredients | Measure | | Carbohydrates (gm.) | Protein (gm.) | Fat (gm.) |
|---|---|---|---|---|---|
| Ground beef | 1½ | pounds | | 125 | 90 |
| Golden mushroom soup | 1 | can | 20.4 | 8.7 | 10.5 |
| Dry bread crumbs | ½ | cup | 30 | 4 | |
| Onion, chopped | ¼ | cup | 3.5 | 1 | |
| Egg, slightly beaten | 1 | | | 7 | 5 |
| Salt | ½ | teaspoon | | | |
| Pepper | | generous dash | | | |
| Potatoes, mashed | 2 | cups | 60 | 8 | |
| Water | ¼ | cup | | | |
| | | | 113.9 | 153.7 | 105.5 |
| Calories: 1 serving—346 | | | 20 | 26 | 18 |

Mix thoroughly beef, ½ cup soup, bread crumbs, onion, egg, salt, and pepper. Shape firmly into loaf and place in shallow baking pan. Bake at 350 degrees 1 hour. Frost loaf with potatoes and bake 15 minutes more. Blend remaining soup, water and 1 tablespoon of drippings. Heat and serve with loaf.

Servings: 6
Exchange per serving: 3 meat, 1½ bread, 1 fat

# Spaghetti Meat Loaf

| Ingredients | Measure | | Carbohy-drates (gm.) | Protein (gm.) | Fat (gm.) |
|---|---|---|---|---|---|
| Ground beef | 1½ | pounds | | 125 | 90 |
| Onion, chopped | ½ | cup | 7 | 2 | |
| Egg, slightly beaten | 1 | | | 7 | 5 |
| Salt, seasoned | 1 | teaspoon | | | |
| Spaghetti in tomato sauce | 1 | 15¼-ounce can | 46.8 | 9.6 | 2.1 |
| | | | 53.8 | 143.6 | 97.1 |
| Calories: 1 serving—258 | | | 9 | 24 | 14 |

Toss together all ingredients with a fork until combined. Turn into lightly greased loaf pan and bake, uncovered, 1 hour at 350 degrees.

Servings: 6
Exchange per serving: 3 meat, 1 bread

# Ribbon Meat Loaf

| Ingredients | Measure | Carbohydrates (gm.) | Protein (gm.) | Fat (gm.) |
|---|---|---|---|---|
| Ground beef | 1½ pounds | | 125 | 90 |
| Egg | 1 | | 7 | 5 |
| Catsup | 2 tablespoons | 9.8 | .8 | |
| Salt | 2 teaspoons | | | |
| Dry mustard | 1 teaspoon | | | |
| Pepper | dash | | | |
| Onion, chopped | ¼ cup | 3.5 | 1 | |
| Margarine | 2 tablespoons | | | 30 |
| Lemon juice | ½ teaspoon | | | |
| Mushroom stems and pieces | 1 4-ounce can | | | |
| Chopped parsley | 2 tablespoons | | | |
| Thyme | ¼ teaspoon | | | |
| Soft bread crumbs | 4 slices | 60 | 8 | |
| | | 73.3 | 141.8 | 125 |

Calories: 1 serving—323.2                                    12.2   23.6   20

Combine beef, egg, catsup, 1½ teaspoons salt, mustard, and pepper in a large bowl; mix lightly with a fork just until blended. Saute onion in margarine just until soft; remove from heat. Stir in lemon juice, mushroom, parsley, ½ teaspoon salt, and thyme. Pour over bread crumbs; toss lightly to mix. Spoon half of meat mixture in greased loaf pan; top with stuffing; pat remaining meat mixture over stuffing to cover completely. Bake at 350 degrees for 1 hour.

Servings: 6
Exchange per serving: 3 meat, 1 bread, 1 fat

# Cheese-Filled Meatloaf

| Ingredients | Measure | Carbohydrates (gm.) | Protein (gm.) | Fat (gm.) |
|---|---|---|---|---|
| Ground beef | 1½ pounds | | 125 | 90 |
| Tomato sauce | 16 ounces | 56 | 16 | |
| Egg, lightly beaten | 1 | | 7 | 5 |
| Dry bread crumbs | ½ cup | 30 | 4 | |
| Onion, finely chopped | ¼ cup | 3.5 | 1 | |
| Salt | 1 teaspoon | | | |
| Pepper | ¼ teaspoon | | | |
| Thyme | ¼ teaspoon | | | |
| American processed cheese | 6 ½-ounce slices | | 21 | 15 |
| | | 89.5 | 174 | 110 |
| Calories: 1 serving—281.4 | | 11.1 | 21 | 17 |

Combine beef, half the tomato sauce, egg, bread crumbs, onion, and seasonings. Place half the mixture in loaf pan. Arrange 4 cheese slices on top and pack remaining meat evenly over the cheese layer. Turn out onto a shallow baking pan. Cut remaining cheese slices in strips and arrange on top of loaf. Bake at 350 degrees for 40 minutes. Pour remaining tomato sauce over loaf. Bake 30 minutes longer.

Servings: 8
Exchange per serving: 3 meat, 1 fruit

# Favorite Meat Loaf

| Ingredients | Measure | Carbohy-drates (gm.) | Pro-tein (gm.) | Fat (gm.) |
|---|---|---|---|---|
| Eggs | 2 | | 14 | 10 |
| Catsup | ⅓ cup | 24.5 | 2 | |
| Warm water | ¾ cup | | | |
| Onion soup mix | 1 envelope | 30 | 4 | |
| Dry bread crumbs | 1½ cups | 90 | 12 | |
| Ground beef | 2 pounds | | 168 | 120 |
| | | 144.5 | 200 | 130 |
| Calories: 1 serving—325 | | 18 | 25 | 17 |

Beat eggs lightly in large bowl. Stir in catsup, water, and soup mix. Add bread crumbs and beef. Pack into loaf pan. Bake at 350 degrees for 1 hour.

Servings: 8
Exchange per serving: 3 meat, 1 bread, ½ vegetable B

# Pizza Burger

| Ingredients | Measure | | Carbohydrates (gm.) | Protein (gm.) | Fat (gm.) |
|---|---|---|---|---|---|
| Tomato soup | 1 | 10½-ounce can | 36.9 | 4.2 | 4.8 |
| Ground beef | 1½ | pounds | | 126 | 90 |
| Dry bread crumbs | ¼ | cup | 15 | 2 | |
| Minced onion | ¼ | cup | 3.5 | 1 | |
| Egg, slightly beaten | 1 | | | 7 | 5 |
| Salt | 1 | teaspoon | | | |
| Crushed oregano | ⅛ | teaspoon | | | |
| Mozzarella cheese, sliced | 4 | ounces | | 28 | 20 |
| | | | 55.4 | 168.2 | 119.8 |

Calories: 1 serving—327.9

|  | 9.2 | 28 | 19.9 |
|---|---|---|---|

Combine ¼ cup soup with beef, bread crumbs, onion, egg, salt, and oregano. Place a square of foil on cookie sheet and pat meat mixture out on foil into a 10-inch circle forming 1-inch standing rim around edge. Spread remaining soup over meat. Top with cheese and more oregano. Can also add mushrooms. Bake at 450 degrees for 15 minutes or until done.

Servings: 6
Exchange per serving: 4 meat, 1 fruit

# Hasty Italian Pizza Supper

| Ingredients | Measure | Carbohydrates (gm.) | Protein (gm.) | Fat (gm.) |
|---|---|---|---|---|
| English muffins, split | 2 | 30 | 4 | 5 |
| Tomato, sliced | 1 | | | |
| Ground beef | ½ pound | | 42 | 30 |
| Onion, chopped | ½ tablespoon | | | |
| Garlic, minced | ¼ teaspoon | | | |
| Salt | ½ teaspoon | | | |
| Mozzarella cheese | 4 1-ounce sliced | | 28 | 20 |
| Basil | ⅛ teaspoon | | | |
| Oregano | ⅛ teaspoon | | | |
| | | 30 | 74 | 55 |
| Calories: 1 serving—228.8 | | 7.5 | 18.2 | 14 |

Toast split muffins lightly. Place halves on cookie sheet and top each with tomato slice. Combine beef, onion, garlic and salt and blend well. Spread ¼ on top of each tomato slice. Top with slice of cheese and sprinkle with basil and oregano. Bake 15 minutes at 400 degrees.

Servings: 4
Exchange per serving: 2 meat, ½ bread, 1 fat

# Pizza Buns

| Ingredients | Measure | | Carbohydrates (gm.) | Protein (gm.) | Fat (gm.) |
|---|---|---|---|---|---|
| Ground beef | 1 | pound | | 84 | 60 |
| Tomato paste | 1 | can | 42 | 12 | |
| Salt | ½ | teaspoon | | | |
| Pepper | | few grains | | | |
| Hamburger buns | 8 | | 180 | 24 | |
| Mushroom stems and pieces | 1 | 4-ounce can | | | |
| Oregano | | as desired | | | |
| Mozzarella cheese, sliced | 8 | ounces | | 56 | 40 |
| | | | 222 | 176 | 100 |
| Calories: 1 serving—311.3 | | | 27.7 | 22 | 12.5 |

Lightly brown meat in skillet. Stir in tomato paste, salt, and pepper. Toast buns slightly on cut sides. Spoon beef mixture on bottom half of buns; top with a spoonful of mushrooms, a sprinkle of oregano, and a slice of cheese. Place top of bun over filling. Wrap each bun securely in heavy foil. Heat in oven at 400 degrees for 15 minutes.

Servings: 8
Exchange per serving: 2½ meat, 2 bread

# Chili Con Carne

| Ingredients | Measure | | Carbohydrates (gm.) | Protein (gm.) | Fat (gm.) |
|---|---|---|---|---|---|
| Ground beef | 1 | pound | | 84 | 60 |
| Onion, chopped | ¼ | cup | 3.5 | 1 | |
| Clove garlic, minced | 1 | | | | |
| Tomato sauce | 8 | ounces | 28 | 8 | |
| Kidney beans | 2 | cups | 79.2 | 29.2 | 2 |
| Liquid (from beans and water) | 2 | cups | | | |
| Chili powder | 2 | teaspoons | | | |
| Tabasco | ¼ | teaspoon | | | |
| Salt | 1 | teaspoon | | | |
| | | | 110.7 | 122.2 | 62 |

Calories: 1 serving—371.9       27.6   30.5   15.5

Brown meat, onion, and garlic, stirring to break meat into pieces. Add remaining ingredients. Cook over low heat 1 to 1½ hours, uncovered. Stir occasionally. Add water, if needed.

Servings: 4
Exchange per serving: 3 meat, 1 bread, 1 skim milk, or 4 meat, 1 bread, 1 fruit (add 1 fat exchange to daily diet)

# Potato Burgers

| Ingredients | Measure | | Carbohydrates (gm.) | Protein (gm.) | Fat (gm.) |
|---|---|---|---|---|---|
| Potatoes, cooked and diced | 1½ | cups | 45 | 6 | |
| Salt | 1 | teaspoon | | | |
| Pepper | ¼ | teaspoon | | | |
| Grated onion | 1 | tablespoon | | | |
| Chopped parsley | 1 | tablespoon | | | |
| Tomato sauce | 8 | ounces | 28 | 8 | |
| Ground beef | 1 | pound | | 84 | 60 |
| | | | 73 | 98 | 60 |
| Calories: 1 serving—303 | | | 18 | 24 | 15 |

Brown beef in skillet. Combine potatoes, salt, pepper, onion, parsley, and ¼ cup tomato sauce. Add to meat and brown 5 minutes. Pour remaining tomato sauce over all, cover, and simmer 10 minutes.

Servings: 4
Exchange per serving: 3 meat, 1 bread, ⅓ fruit

# Hobo Stew

| Ingredients | Measure | Carbohydrates (gm.) | Protein (gm.) | Fat (gm.) |
|---|---|---|---|---|
| Onion, thinly sliced | 1 cup | 14 | 4 | |
| Olive oil | ¼ cup | | | 60 |
| Ground beef | 1¼ pounds | | 105 | 75 |
| Red kidney beans, drained | 1 1-pound can | 39.6 | 14.6 | 1 |
| Worcestershire sauce | 1 tablespoon | | | |
| Whole kernel corn, drained | 1 1-pound can | 31.8 | 4.4 | 1.2 |
| Tomatoes | 1 32-ounce can | | | |
| Tomato sauce | 16 ounces | 56 | 16 | |
| Basil | as desired | | | |
| Dry mustard | as desired | | | |
| Salt | as desired | | | |
| Pepper | as desired | | | |
| | | 141.4 | 144 | 137.2 |
| Calories: 1 serving—394.3 | | 23.5 | 24 | 22.7 |

Cook onion in oil until golden. Add beef and cook, stirring with fork to break up meat, until browned. Add remaining ingredients and mix well. Cover and simmer 15 to 20 minutes.

Servings: 6
Exchange per serving: 1 bread, 3 meat, 1½ fat, ½ vegetable B

# Spaghetti and Meatballs

| Ingredients | Measure | Carbohydrates (gm.) | Protein (gm.) | Fat (gm.) |
|---|---|---|---|---|
| Onions, chopped | 2 | 14 | 4 | |
| Olive oil | 2 tablespoons | | | 30 |
| Tomatoes | 1 29-ounce can | | | |
| Tomato sauce | 8 ounces | 28 | 8 | |
| Chopped parsley | ¼ cup | | | |
| Garlic salt | 2½ teaspoons | | | |
| Pepper | ¼ teaspoon | | | |
| Crushed red pepper | ¼ teaspoon | | | |
| Tomato paste | 1 can | 42 | 12 | |
| Meatballs (recipe below) | | 22 | 116 | 80 |
| | | 106 | 140 | 110 |

Calories: 1 serving—328.3     17.6   23.3   18.3

Cook onions in oil until yellowed. Add tomatoes, bring to a boil, and simmer, uncovered, for 20 minutes. Add remaining ingredients and simmer uncovered 2 hours longer, stirring occasionally. Serve over cooked spaghetti allowing ½ cup spaghetti, 2 meatballs, and 1/6 sauce per person.

Servings: 6

Exchange per serving: 2 bread, 3 meat, ½ fat, ¼ fruit

# Meatballs

| Ingredients | Measure | | Carbohydrates (gm.) | Protein (gm.) | Fat (gm. |
|---|---|---|---|---|---|
| Ground beef | 1¼ | pound | | 105 | 75 |
| Onions, minced | 1 | | 7 | 2 | |
| Chopped parsley | ¼ | cup | | | |
| Dry bread crumbs | ¼ | cup | 15 | 2 | |
| Egg | 1 | | | 7 | 5 |
| Garlic salt | 2 | teaspoons | | | |
| Pepper | ½ | teaspoon | | | |
| Oregano | ½ | teaspoon | | | |
| | | | 22 | 116 | 80 |
| Calories: 1 serving—207.4 | | | 3.6 | 19 | 13 |

Combine all ingredients and shape into 12 balls.

Servings: 6 (2 meatballs each)
Exchange per serving: 3 meat, ⅓ fruit

# Spaghetti Amore

| Ingredients | Measure | Carbohydrates (gm.) | Protein (gm.) | Fat (gm.) |
|---|---|---|---|---|
| Ground beef | 1 pound | | 84 | 60 |
| Onion, chopped | ½ cup | 7 | 2 | |
| Oil | 1 tablespoon | | | 15 |
| Cream of mushroom soup | 1 10½-ounce can | 22.5 | 5.1 | 26.1 |
| Tomato soup | 1 10½-ounce can | 36.9 | 4.2 | 4.8 |
| Water | 1 soup can | | | |
| Cheese, shredded sharp processed | 1 cup | | 56 | 40 |
| Spaghetti, cooked, drained | ½ pound | 120 | 16 | |
| | | 186.4 | 167.3 | 145.9 |
| Calories: 1 serving—453.9 | | 31 | 27.8 | 24.3 |

Lightly brown beef and onion in oil. Add soups and water; heat. Add ½ cup cheese and spaghetti. Pour into 3-quart casserole, top with remaining ½ cup cheese; bake at 350 degrees for 30 minutes.

Servings: 6

Exchange per serving: 2 bread, 4 meat, 1 fat

# Lasagne

| Ingredients | Measure | Carbohydrates (gm.) | Protein (gm.) | Fat (gm.) |
|---|---|---|---|---|
| Olive or salad oil | 2 tablespoons | | | 30 |
| Onion, chopped | 1 | 7 | 2 | |
| Ground beef | 1 pound | | 84 | 60 |
| Garlic salt | 2 teaspoons | | | |
| Pepper | ¼ teaspoon | | | |
| Tomato paste | 2 6-ounce cans | 84 | 14 | |
| Hot water | 3 cups | | | |
| Lasagne noodles, cooked, drained | ½ pound | 120 | 16 | |
| Cottage cheese | ½ pound | | 28 | 20 |
| Mozzarella cheese | ½ pound | | 56 | 40 |
| | | 211 | 200 | 150 |

Calories: 1 serving—373.5      26.3   25   18.7

Saute onion in oil. Add beef and cook and stir until crumbly. Mix in garli
salt, pepper, and tomato paste blended with hot water. Simmer, uncovered
30 minutes. In shallow baking dish put a thin layer of sauce, half the lasagne
all the cottage cheese, and thin slice of mozzarella. Repeat with half the
remaining sauce, the lasagne, the last of the sauce, and mozzarella. Bake a
350 degrees for 30 minutes. Leave out of oven for 15 minutes; then cut into
squares.

Servings: 8
Exchange per serving: 2 bread, 3 meat, 1 fat

# Six-Layer Dinner

| Ingredients | Measure | Carbohydrates (gm.) | Protein (gm.) | Fat (gm.) |
|---|---|---|---|---|
| Potatoes, sliced, raw | 4 | 60 | 8 | |
| Ground beef | 1 pound | | 84 | 60 |
| Onions, sliced | 2 cups | 28 | 8 | |
| Corn, drained | 1⅓ cups | 60 | 8 | |
| Tomatoes | 16-ounce can | | | |
| | | 148 | 108 | 60 |
| Calories: 1 serving—391 | | 37 | 27 | 15 |

In a casserole, layer potatoes, then beef, onions, corn, and tomatoes. Season layers with 2 teaspoons salt and ¼ teaspoon pepper. Bake at 350 degrees for 2 hours.

Servings: 4

Exchange per serving: 3 meat, 2 bread, 1 vegetable B, 1 vegetable A

# Stuffed Cabbage Rolls

| Ingredients | Measure | Carbohydrates (gm.) | Protein (gm.) | Fat (gm.) |
|---|---|---|---|---|
| Cabbage leaves | 12 large | | | |
| Ground beef | 1¼ pound | | 105 | 75 |
| Salt | 2 teaspoons | | | |
| Pepper | ½ teaspoon | | | |
| Rice, cooked | 1 cup | 30 | 4 | |
| Onion, chopped | 1 | 7 | 2 | |
| Egg | 1 | | 7 | 5 |
| Poultry seasoning | ½ teaspoon | | | |
| Tomato sauce | 16-ounces | 48 | 16 | |
| Water | ¼ cup | | | |
| Lemon juice | 1 tablespoon | | | |
| | | 85 | 134 | 80 |

Calories: 1 serving—288          14      22      16

Cover cabbage with boiling water and let stand 5 minutes. Peel off 12 nice leaves. Combine beef, salt, pepper, rice, onion, egg, and poultry seasoning. Place equal portions in center of each leaf; fold sides of leaf over meat and roll up. Place in small casserole. Combine water, lemon juice, and tomato sauce and pour over rolls. Cover. Bake at 350 degrees for 1 hour.

Servings: 6 (2 rolls each)
Exchange per serving: 3 meat, 1 bread

# Meat Patty With Cheese Sauce

| Ingredients | Measure | Carbohydrates (gm.) | Protein (gm.) | Fat (gm.) |
|---|---|---|---|---|
| Ground beef | 1 pound | | 84 | 60 |
| Cream of celery soup, undiluted | 1 10½-ounce can | 19.2 | 4.2 | 11.7 |
| Grated cheese | 4 ounces | | 28 | 20 |
| | | 19.2 | 116.2 | 91.7 |
| Calories: 1 serving—341.3 | | 4.8 | 29 | 22.9 |

Form beef into 4 patties and broil on both sides. Heat soup in double boiler and stir in cheese. As soon as cheese melts, pour ¼ sauce over each patty and serve at once.

Servings: 4
Exchange per serving: 4 meat, ½ fruit

# Oven Beef Bake

| Ingredients | Measure | Carbohydrates (gm.) | Protein (gm.) | Fat (gm.) |
|---|---|---|---|---|
| Elbow macaroni, cooked and drained | 8-ounces | 120 | 16 | |
| Carrots, sliced | 1-pound can | 28 | 8 | |
| Mushrooms, sliced | 1 6-ounce can | | | |
| Ground beef | 2 pounds | | 168 | 120 |
| Onion, chopped | 1 | 7 | 2 | |
| Celery, thinly sliced | 2 cups | | | |
| Margarine | 4 tablespoons | | | 60 |
| Flour | 5 tablespoons | 55.8 | 7.5 | |
| Salt | 1 teaspoon | | | |
| Pepper | ¼ teaspoon | | | |
| Condensed beef broth | 1 10½-ounce can | | | |
| | | 210.8 | 201.5 | 180 |

Calories: 1 serving—416.6      27.3   25.1   23

Drain liquids from carrots and mushrooms and set aside. Combine vegetables with macaroni in a greased 12-cup baking dish. Brown ground meat and stir into vegetable mixture. Saute onion and celery in margarine until golden in same frying pan; sprinkle with flour, salt, and pepper, then stir in. Cook, stirring constantly, just until bubbly. Combine beef broth with saved vegetable juices; add water, if needed, to make 3 cups; stir into onion mixture. Continue cooking and stirring until sauce thickens and boils 1 minute. Pour over meat and vegetables; cover. Bake at 350 for 1 hour.

Servings: 8
Exchange per serving: 2 bread, 3 meat, 1½ fat

# Chapter X

# Poultry

RECIPE FOR

# Chicken Paella

| Ingredients | Measure | Carbohy-drates (gm.) | Pro-tein (gm.) | Fat (gm.) |
|---|---|---|---|---|
| Onions, sliced | 1 medium | 7 | 2 | |
| Green pepper, chopped | ½ cup | | | |
| Monosodium glutamate | 2 teaspoons | | | |
| Boiling water | 2½ cups | | | |
| Converted rice | 1 cup | 120 | 16 | |
| Margarine | ¼ cup | | | 60 |
| Mushrooms, sliced | 1 cup | | | |
| Green peas, frozen | 1 10-ounce package | 36 | 15 | .9 |
| Chicken, diced and cooked | 2 cups | | 112 | 80 |
| Tomato, cut in wedges | 1 medium | | | |
| | | 163 | 145 | 140.9 |

Calories: 1 serving—420     27   24   24

Melt margarine in pan; sauté onion and green pepper; add mushrooms and sauté until tender. Add water, rice, and monosodium glutamate. Cover pan with lid and place in oven at 350 degrees for 25 minutes. Stir in peas and half the chicken. Arrange remaining chicken and tomato on top. Cover and return to oven for 15 minutes.

Servings: 6
Exchange per serving: 3 meat, 2 bread, 2 fat

# Chicken Fricasee

| Ingredients | Measure | | Carbohy-drates (gm.) | Pro-tein (gm.) | Fat (gm.) |
|---|---|---|---|---|---|
| Chicken broiler-fryer | 3½ | pounds | | 189 | 135 |
| Onion, chopped | ½ | cup | | | |
| Carrot, pared and sliced thinly | 1 | | | | |
| Celery, sliced thinly | 1 | stalk | | | |
| Salt | 2 | teaspoons | | | |
| Peppercorns | 6 | whole | | | |
| Bay leaf | 1 | | | | |
| Water | | | | | |
| Margarine | 6 | tablespoons | | | 90 |
| Flour | 6 | tablespoons | 67.2 | 9 | 2.4 |
| Peas, frozen | 1 | 10-ounce package | 36 | 15 | .9 |
| Corn meal dumplings (recipe below) | | | 131 | 19.6 | 37.5 |
| | | | 234.2 | 232.6 | 265.8 |
| Calories: 1 serving—530.8 | | | 29 | 29 | 33.2 |

Combine first 7 ingredients in dutch oven with water to cover. Heat to boiling, cover, and simmer 2 hours, or until chicken is tender. Remove and set aside. Strain broth into 4-cup measure (add water, if necessary, to make 4 cups). Press vegetables through sieve into broth. Melt margarine in same kettle; stir in flour; cook, stirring constantly, just until bubbly. Stir in 4 cups broth; continue cooking and stirring until gravy thickens and boils 1 minute. Season to taste with salt and pepper. Place chicken in gravy, add peas, and heat slowly to boiling while preparing corn meal dumplings. Drop batter in 8 mounds on top of boiling chicken; cover. Cook until puffy light, about 20 minutes.

Servings: 8
Exchange per serving: 3 meat, 2 bread, 3 fat (including dumplings)

# Corn Meal Dumplings

| Ingredients | Measure | Carbohydrates (gm.) | Protein (gm.) | Fat (gm.) |
|---|---|---|---|---|
| Flour, sifted | ¾ cup | 57 | 8 | .6 |
| Baking powder | 1½ teaspoons | | | |
| Salt | ½ teaspoon | | | |
| Yellow corn meal | ½ cup | 66 | 6.6 | .9 |
| Milk | ⅔ cup | 8 | 5 | 6 |
| Vegetable oil | 2 tablespoons | | | 30 |
| | | 131 | 19.6 | 37.5 |
| Calories: 1 serving—120 | | 17 | 2.4 | 4.7 |

Place dry ingredients in a bowl. Combine milk and oil in 1-cup measure and add all at once to dry ingredients. Stir just until evenly moist. (Dough will be soft.)

Servings: 8
Exchange per serving: 1 bread, 1 fat

# Chicken Cacciatora

| Ingredients | Measure | Carbohydrates (gm.) | Protein (gm.) | Fat (gm.) |
|---|---|---|---|---|
| Chicken breasts, frying | 3½ pounds | | 189 | 135 |
| Olive oil | 2 tablespoons | | | 30 |
| Garlic | 1 clove | | | |
| Oregano | 1 teaspoon | | | |
| Salt | as desired | | | |
| Pepper | as desired | | | |
| Sliced mushrooms | 1½ cups | | | |
| Stewed tomatoes | 1 16-ounce can | | | |
| | | | 189 | 165 |
| Calories: 1 serving—274.4 | | | 23.6 | 20 |

Brown chicken in oil with garlic. Before turning, sprinkle with oregano, salt, and pepper. Remove garlic. Add mushrooms, brown lightly. Add tomatoes. Cover and simmer 30 minutes. Uncover; continue cooking until sauce is reduced to consistency desired and chicken is very tender. Garnish with parsley.

Servings: 8
Exchange per serving: 3½ meat, ½ fat

# Oven Crisp Chicken

| Ingredients | Measure | | Carbohydrates (gm.) | Protein (gm.) | Fat (gm.) |
|---|---|---|---|---|---|
| Chicken, broiler-fryer | 3½ | pounds | | 189 | 135 |
| Onion soup mix | 2 | packets | 60 | 8 | |
| Dry bread crumbs | 1 | cup | 60 | 8 | |
| Salt | 1 | teaspoon | | | |
| Pepper | ⅛ | teaspoon | | | |
| | | | 120 | 205 | 135 |

| | Carbohydrates | Protein | Fat |
|---|---|---|---|
| Calories: 1 serving—315.6 | 15 | 25.6 | 16.8 |

Combine soup mix, bread crumbs, salt, and pepper in a paper bag. Shake chicken pieces, a few at a time, in mixture to coat well. Place, not touching, in a single layer in a buttered shallow baking pan. Bake at 350 degrees for 1 hour, or until chicken is tender and richly browned.

Servings: 8
Exchange per serving: 1 bread, 3½ meat

# Apricot Chicken

| Ingredients | Measure | Car-bohy-drates (gm.) | Pro-tein (gm.) | Fat (gm.) |
|---|---|---|---|---|
| Apricot jelly, low calorie | 1 8-ounce jar | 15 | | |
| Onion soup mix | 1 package | 30 | 4 | |
| Russian dressing, low calorie | 1 8-ounce jar | 56 | | 1 |
| Chicken, broiler-fryer | 3½ pounds | | 189 | 135 |
| | | 101 | 193 | 136 |
| Calories: 1 serving—212.6 | | 12.5 | 24 | 17 |

Combine jelly, soup mix and dressing. Pour over chicken and marinade 24 hours. Bake uncovered for 1½ hours at 350 degrees.

Servings: 8
Exchange per serving: 3 meat, 1 bread

# Man's Barbecued Chicken

| Ingredients | Measure | | Carbohydrates (gm.) | Protein (gm.) | Fat (gm.) |
|---|---|---|---|---|---|
| Garlic salt | | as desired | | | |
| Pepper | | as desired | | | |
| Tomato juice | 1½ | cups | | | |
| Cayenne pepper | ¼ | teaspoon | | | |
| Dry mustard | ¼ | teaspoon | | | |
| Bay leaf | 1 | | | | |
| Worcestershire sauce | 4½ | teaspoons | | | |
| Cider vinegar | ¾ | cup | | | |
| Artificial sweetener | = 1 | teaspoon sugar | | | |
| Margarine or salad oil | 3 | tablespoons | | | 45 |
| Chicken, broiler-fryer | 3½ | pounds | | 189 | 135 |
| Onions | 1½ | | 10 | 3 | |
| | | | 10 | 192 | 180 |

Calories: 1 serving—304.5  ·  1.5  24  22.5

Day before or early in day make barbecue sauce: combine 2 teaspoons garlic salt, ¼ teaspoon pepper, tomato juice, cayenne, mustard, bay leaf, Worcestershire, vinegar, artificial sweetener, and margarine. Simmer, uncovered, 10 minutes, then refrigerate. About 1½ hours before serving arrange chicken, skin side up, in shallow pan. Sprinkle lightly with salt and pepper. Slice onions and layer over chicken. Pour on sauce. Bake, uncovered, at 350 degrees for 30 minutes, basting often; turn, bake 45 minutes longer, basting often.

Servings: 8
Exchange per serving: 3½ meat, 1 fat

# Weight Watcher's Chicken With Pineapple

| Ingredients | Measure | Carbohydrates (gm.) | Protein (gm.) | Fat (gm.) |
|---|---|---|---|---|
| Chicken, broiler-fryer | 3½ pounds | | 189 | 135 |
| Soy sauce | ¼ cup | | | |
| Monosodium glutamate | 1 teaspoon | | | |
| Lemon juice | 2 tablespoons | | | |
| Clove garlic, crushed | 1 | | | |
| Sliced pineapple, dietetic | 1 8-ounce can | 40 | | |
| | | 40 | 189 | 135 |

Calories: 1 serving—265.2      5   23.6   16.8

Mix soy sauce, lemon juice, and garlic. Place chicken in shallow pan; sprinkle with monosodium glutamate; pour mixture over and let stand for few hours, turning once or twice. Remove chicken to broiling rack (reserve marinade). Broil chicken 6 inches from fire for 20 minutes until charred. Turn. Drain Pineapple (reserve juice) and place slices in pan under rack. Spoon marinade over pineapple. Continue broiling until chicken is charred and tender—about 10 minutes. Remove chicken and pineapple to serving dish. Remove rack, add pineapple juice to marinade, and stir over low heat. Serve sauce on side. (Can be spooned over cooked rice as a side dish.)

Servings: 8
Exchange per serving: ½ fruit, 3 meat

# Chicken Chow Mein

| Ingredients | Measure | | Carbohydrates (gm.) | Protein (gm.) | Fat (gm.) |
|---|---|---|---|---|---|
| Chicken bouillon cube | 1 | | | | |
| Artificial sweetener | = | 2 tablespoons sugar | | | |
| Water | ¾ | cup | | | |
| Soy sauce | ¼ | cup | | | |
| Chicken, diced and cooked | 3 | cups | | 168 | 120 |
| Chinese vegetables | 1 | 16-ounce can | | | |
| Chinese noodles | 1 | can | 45 | 6 | 20 |
| Rice, cooked | 2 | cups | 60 | 8 | |
| | | | 105 | 182 | 140 |
| Calories: 1 serving—399.7 | | | 17.5 | 30 | 23.3 |

Combine bouillon cube, artificial sweetener, water, and soy sauce. Bring to a boil and simmer 5 minutes. Heat chicken in sauce. Heat Chinese vegetables. Combine with chicken and serve over rice and Chinese noodles.

Servings: 6
Exchange per serving: 4 meat, 1 fruit, 1 vegetable B, ½ fat

# Chicken Pie—Using Leftover Chicken

| Ingredients | Measure | Carbohydrates (gm.) | Protein (gm.) | Fat (gm.) |
|---|---|---|---|---|
| Chicken, cooked | 3 cups | | 168 | 120 |
| Potatoes, quartered | 6 | 90 | 12 | |
| Onions, quartered | 4 | 28 | 8 | |
| Carrots, sliced | 4 | | | |
| Parsley, chopped | 2 tablespoons | | | |
| Margarine | 3 tablespoons | | | 45 |
| Flour | 2 tablespoons | 22.4 | 3 | |
| Salt | ½ teaspoon | | | |
| Pepper | ⅛ teaspoon | | | |
| Chicken broth | 1 13¾-ounce can | | | |
| Refrigerated biscuits | 1 8-ounce package | 150 | 20 | |
| | | 290.4 | 211 | 165 |
| Calories: 1 serving—583.1 | | 48.4 | 35 | 27.5 |

In large covered saucepan cook potatoes, onions and carrots in 2 cups water for 15 minutes. Drain well. Mix with chicken and parsley in 3-quart baking dish. Blend flour, salt and pepper in 2 tablespoons melted margarine. Gradually stir in chicken broth and cook, stirring constantly, until sauce thickens and comes to a boil. Pour over chicken-vegetable mixture. Flatten biscuits and arrange over top of mixture. Brush with 1 tablespoon melted margarine. Bake 45 minutes at 350 degrees.

Servings: 6
Exchange per serving: 4 meat, 3 bread, 1½ fat

# CHAPTER XI

# Fish

BIRDSEYE FISH

|  |  | Carbohydrate | Protein | Fat |
|---|---|---|---|---|
| Fillets, cod | 2 | 0 | 18.8 | .4 |
| Fillets, flounder | 2 | 0 | 16.8 | .6 |
| Fillets, haddock | 2 | 0 | 20.8 | . |
| Fillets, perch | 2 | 0 | 21.2 | .9 |
| Fillets, sole | 2 | 0 | 20.8 | .2 |
| Fish bites | ½ package | 24.6 | 11.2 | 13.8 |
| Fish sticks, cod | 5 sticks | 29.1 | 15.1 | 10.7 |
| Fish sticks, haddock | 5 sticks | 29.1 | 16.2 | 10.5 |
| Scallops, sea | ½ package | 25.4 | 12.3 | 6.0 |
| Steak, halibut | ½ steak | 0 | 21.2 | 6.0 |

# Scandinavian Fish Bake

| Ingredients | Measure | Car-bohy-drates (gm.) | Pro-tein (gm.) | Fat (gm.) |
|---|---|---|---|---|
| Cod, haddock, or flounder fillets | 1 pound | | 84 | |
| Flour | 4 tablespoons | 44.8 | 6 | |
| Salt | 2 teaspoons | | | |
| Pepper | ¼ teaspoon | | | |
| Milk, skim | 1 cup | 12 | 8 | |
| Dry bread crumbs | ½ cup | 30 | 4 | |
| Margarine, melted | 2 tablespoons | | | 30 |
| Chopped parsley | 1 tablespoon | | | |
| Sour cream | ½ cup | | | 20 |
| | | 86.8 | 102 | 50 |
| Calories: 1 serving—301.3 | | 21.7 | 25.5 | 12.5 |

Cut fillets into serving pieces and coat with mixture of flour, salt, and pepper. Arrange in single layer in baking dish and pour milk over. Bake at 350 degrees for 45 minutes. Mix crumbs with margarine in a small bowl. Stir parsley into sour cream in another bowl. Remove fish from oven; spoon sour cream over, then buttered crumbs. Bake 10 minutes longer, or until sour cream is set.

Servings: 4

Exchange per serving: 1 bread, 1 vegetable B, 3 meat (add ½ fat to daily diet)

# Broiled Cod Piquant

| Ingredients | Measure | Carbohydrates (gm.) | Protein (gm.) | Fat (gm.) |
|---|---|---|---|---|
| Cod fillets | 1 pound | | 84 | |
| Mayonnaise | 4 teaspoons | | | 20 |
| Salt | as desired | | | |
| Pepper | as desired | | | |
| Dry bread crumbs | ¼ cup | 15 | 2 | |
| | | 15 | 86 | 20 |
| Calories: 1 serving—145.8 | | 3.7 | 21.5 | 5 |

Spread fish with mayonnaise. Sprinkle with salt and pepper. Broil 3 inches from fire for 8 minutes. Sprinkle with crumbs and broil 2 or 3 minutes or until browned.

Servings: 4
Exchange per serving: 3 meat, ⅓ fruit (add 2 fat exchanges to daily diet)

# Tomato Glazed Fillets

| Ingredients | Measure | Car-<br>bohy-<br>drates<br>(gm.) | Pro-<br>tein<br>(gm.) | Fat<br>(gm.) |
|---|---|---|---|---|
| Vegetable or olive oil | 2 tablespoons | | | 30 |
| Onion, thinly sliced | 1 | 7 | 2 | |
| Mushroom, stems and pieces | 1 4-ounce can | | | |
| Cod or haddock fillets | 1 pound | | 84 | |
| Garlic salt | ½ teaspoon | | | |
| Salt | 1 teaspoon | | | |
| Grated lemon rind | ½ teaspoon | | | |
| Ground dill seed | ¼ teaspoon | | | |
| Tomato juice | 2 cups | | | |
| Flour | 2 tablespoons | 22.4 | 3 | |
| Lemon juice | 2 tablespoons | | | |
| Artificial sweetener | = 2 tablespoons sugar | | | |
| Chopped parsley | 1 tablespoon | | | |
| | | 29.4 | 89 | 30 |
| Calories: 1 serving—184.7 | | 7.3 | 22 | 7.5 |

Saute onion in oil until tender. Add mushrooms. Arrange fillets over vegetables. Sprinkle with garlic salt, salt, lemon rind, and dill seed. Add tomato juice. Cover and cook over moderate heat for 10 minutes, until fish is easily flaked with a fork. Remove fish to heated platter. Blend flour and lemon juice together. Gradually add ½ cup of mixture from skillet. Pour back into skillet, stirring vigorously. Add artificial sweetener; cook over moderate heat, stirring constantly, until thickened. Pour over fish and garnish with parsley.

Servings: 4
Exchange per serving: 3 meat, 1 vegetable B (add 1½ fat to daily diet)

# Fish Fillets in Mushroom Sauce

| Ingredients | Measure | | Carbohydrates (gm.) | Protein (gm.) | Fat (gm.) |
|---|---|---|---|---|---|
| Fresh mushrooms | 1 | cup | | | |
| Margarine | 3 | tablespoons | | | 45 |
| Flour | 2½ | tablespoons | 28 | 3.7 | |
| Salt | ½ | teaspoon | | | |
| Cayenne | | dash | | | |
| Milk, skim | 2 | cups | 24 | 16 | |
| Cod or haddock fillets | 1 | pound | | 84 | |
| Dry bread crumbs | ¼ | cup | 15 | 2 | |
| | | | 67 | 105.7 | 45 |

Calories: 1 serving—271.4    16.7    26.4    11

Wash and slice mushrooms. Saute in margarine for 5 minutes. Add flour and seasonings, mixing to a smooth paste. Add milk gradually, stirring constantly. Cook until thickened. Place fillets in a baking dish and sprinkle with salt. Cover with sauce. Top with bread crumbs. Bake at 375 degrees for 30 minutes.

Servings: 4

Exchange per serving: 1 bread, 4 meat (add 2 fat exchanges to daily diet)

# Yum Yum Sole

| Ingredients | Measure | Carbohydrates (gm.) | Protein (gm.) | Fat (gm.) |
|---|---|---|---|---|
| Sole or flounder fillets | 1 pound | | 84 | |
| Flour | ⅛ cup | 22.4 | 3 | |
| Paprika | 2 teaspoons | | | |
| Salt | 1 teaspoon | | | |
| Salad oil | 1 tablespoon | | | 15 |
| Margarine | ¼ cup | | | 60 |
| Lemon juice | 2 tablespoons | | | |
| Liquid red pepper seasoning | ¼ teaspoon | | | |
| Parsley | few sprigs | | | |
| | | 22.4 | 87 | 75 |

Calories: 1 serving—274.7

|  |  | 5.6 | 21 | 18.7 |
|---|---|---|---|---|

Mix flour, paprika, and salt; coat fish with this mixture. Place in greased shallow baking pan and brush with salad oil. Melt margarine in saucepan; add lemon juice and liquid red pepper seasoning. Broil fish 2 to 3 inches from fire for 8 minutes. Don't turn during broiling. Transfer to a warm platter and pour margarine mixture over the top. Garnish with parsley.

Servings: 4
Exchange per serving: 3 meat, ½ fruit, ½ fat

# Paprika Fish

| Ingredients | Measure | Carbohydrates (gm.) | Protein (gm.) | Fat (gm.) |
|---|---|---|---|---|
| Cod, haddock or flounder fillets | 1 pound | | 84 | |
| Onion, sliced | 1 large | | | |
| Margarine | 2 tablespoons | | | 30 |
| Evaporated milk | ¾ cup | 18 | 12 | 15 |
| Paprika | 1 tablespoon | | | |
| Salt | ¾ teaspoon | | | |
| Pepper | ¼ teaspoon | | | |
| | | 18 | 96 | 45 |
| Calories: 1 serving—213 | | 4.5 | 24 | 11 |

Cook onion in margarine until golden. Put in shallow baking dish. Cut fish in 4 serving pieces and arrange on top of onion. Beat remaining ingredients together lightly and pour over fish. Bake in moderate oven (375 degrees) about 25 minutes.

Servings: 4
Exchange per serving: 3½ meat, ½ fruit (add 1½ fat to daily diet)

# Luncheon Lobster

| Ingredients | Measure | | Carbohydrates (gm.) | Protein (gm.) | Fat (gm.) |
|---|---|---|---|---|---|
| Bay leaf | 1 | | | | |
| Lemon, sliced | 1 | | | | |
| Artificial sweetener | = | 1 teaspoon sugar | | | |
| Salt | 1 | teaspoon | | | |
| Rock lobster tails, frozen | 3 | 8-ounce | .9 | 30 | 3.3 |
| Mushrooms | 1 | 3-ounce can | | | |
| Flour | 1 | tablespoon | 11.2 | 1.5 | |
| Milk, skim | ½ | cup | 6 | 4 | |
| Seasoned salt | ½ | teaspoon | | | |
| Soy sauce | ½ | teaspoon | | | |
| Egg yolk | 1 | | .1 | 2.8 | 5.4 |
| Parmesan cheese, grated | 1 | tablespoon | | | |
| | | | 18.2 | 38.3 | 8.7 |

Calories: 1 serving—101.3      6   12.8   2.9

In saucepan combine 4 cups water, bay leaf, lemon slices, artificial sweetener and salt. Bring to boil. Add lobster tails and boil gently, 10 minutes. Drain.

Drain mushrooms and add water to make ½ cup. Stir into flour in small saucepan. Add milk, seasoned salt and soy sauce. Bring to boil, reduce heat and simmer 3 minutes.

In small bowl beat egg yolk and gradually stir in hot mixture. Return to sauce pan and cook, stirring, just to boiling.

Remove lobster from shells and cut into bite size pieces. (Keep shells intact.) Add lobster and mushrooms to sauce and heat through. Spoon into lobster shells and sprinkle with parmesan cheese. Broil 2 inches from heat 2-3 minutes, until cheese browns.

Servings: 3

Exchange per serving: 1½ meat, ½ bread (add 1 fat to daily allowance)

# Chapter XII

# Tuna and Salmon

# Crown Tuna Casserole

| Ingredients | Measure | Carbohydrates (gm.) | Protein (gm.) | Fat (gm.) |
|---|---|---|---|---|
| Margarine | ¼ cup | | | 60 |
| Onion, chopped | ½ cup | 7 | 2 | |
| Green pepper, chopped | 1 cup | | | |
| Flour | 2 tablespoons | 22.4 | 3 | |
| Tomatoes, canned | 1 1-pound 13-ounce can | | | |
| Worcestershire sauce | 1 tablespoon | | | |
| Dry mustard | 1 teaspoon | | | |
| Salt | ½ teaspoon | | | |
| Artificial sweetener | = ½ teaspoon sugar | | | |
| Pepper | ¼ teaspoon | | | |
| Tuna, water packed | 1 7-ounce can | | 36.4 | 17.2 |
| Buttermilk biscuits, refrigerator | 1 8-ounce can | 150 | 20 | |
| | | 179.4 | 61.4 | 77.2 |
| Calories: 1 serving—277 | | 30 | 10 | 13 |

In hot margarine sauté onion until limp, add green pepper and cook 5 minutes. Stir in flour until blended. Add tomatoes, Worcestershire, mustard, salt, artificial sweetener, and pepper; simmer, covered, 10 minutes. Add tuna and pour into 2½-quart casserole. Cut each biscuit into thirds and arrange with points up on casserole. Bake at 375 degrees for 25 minutes.

Servings: 6
Exchange per serving: 1 meat, 2 bread, 1½ fat

# Salmon Croquettes

| Ingredients | Measure | Carbohydrates (gm.) | Protein (gm.) | Fat (gm.) |
|---|---|---|---|---|
| Salmon, drained | 1 pound can | | 72.8 | 34.4 |
| Dry bread crumbs | ½ cup | 30 | 4 | |
| Eggs | 2 | | 14 | 10 |
| Onion, chopped | 2 tablespoons | | | |
| Salt | as desired | | | |
| Pepper | as desired | | | |
| Water | 2 tablespoons | | | |
| | | 30 | 90.8 | 44.4 |

| | | | | |
|---|---|---|---|---|
| Calories: 1 serving—230.7 | | 7.5 | 25.2 | 11.1 |

Combine salmon, ¼ cup bread crumbs, 1 egg, onion, salt, and pepper. Form into four patties. Beat other egg and add water. Dip patties in egg, coating well, and then in bread crumbs. Brown well on both sides in skillet.

Servings: 4
Exchange per serving: 3 meat, 1 vegetable B (add 1 fat exchange to daily diet)

# Salmon Puffs

| Ingredients | Measure | Carbohydrates (gm.) | Protein (gm.) | Fat (gm.) |
|---|---|---|---|---|
| White bread, in pieces | 4 slices | 60 | 8 | |
| Milk, skim | 1 cup | 12 | 8 | |
| Eggs | 4 | | 28 | 20 |
| Salt | ¼ teaspoon | | | |
| Dry mustard | ½ teaspoon | | | |
| Onion, sliced | 1 | | | |
| Salmon, drained | 1 7¾-ounce can | | 36.4 | 17.2 |
| | | 72 | 80.4 | 37.2 |
| Calories: 1 serving—237.3 | | 18 | 20.1 | 9.3 |

Combine all ingredients in blender. Cover and blend on high speed for 20 seconds. Pour into 4 buttered individual 10-ounce casseroles. Bake at 325 degrees for 30 minutes.

Servings: 4

Exchange per serving: 1 bread, ½ vegetable B, 2 meat

# Salmon Pickle Loaf

| Ingredients | Measure | Car-bohy-drates (gm.) | Pro-tein (gm.) | Fat (gm.) |
|---|---|---|---|---|
| Salmon, drained | 1-pound can | | 72.8 | 34.4 |
| Cream of celery soup | 1 10¾-ounce can | 19.2 | 4.2 | 11.7 |
| Soft bread crumbs | 1½ cups | 90 | 12 | |
| Dill pickles, chopped | ½ cup | | | |
| Eggs, well beaten | 2 | | 14 | 10 |
| Vinegar | 1 tablespoon | | | |
| | | 109.2 | 103 | 56.1 |

Calories: 1 serving—169        13.6    12.9    7

Combine ingredients. Pack into greased loaf pan. Bake at 350 degrees for one hour. Let stand 10 minutes before unmolding.

Servings: 8
Exchange per serving: 2 meat, 1⅓ fruit

# Tuna Jambalaya

| Ingredients | Measure | Carbohydrates (gm.) | Protein (gm.) | Fat (gm.) |
|---|---|---|---|---|
| Margarine | 2 tablespoons | | | 30 |
| Onion, chopped | ½ cup | 7 | 2 | |
| Sliced mushrooms, drained | 1 4-ounce can | | | |
| Tomato soup | 1 10½-ounce can | 36.9 | 4.2 | 4.8 |
| Water | 2 tablespoons | | | |
| Worcestershire sauce | 1 teaspoon | | | |
| Pepper | few grains | | | |
| Tuna, drained, water packed | 1 7-ounce can | | 36.4 | 17.2 |
| Instant rice, prepared according to package directions | 2 cups | 60 | 8 | |
| | | 103.9 | 50.6 | 52 |
| Calories: 1 serving—271 | | 25.9 | 12.6 | 13 |

Melt margarine in skillet. Add onion and mushrooms; cook about 5 minutes over moderate heat, until tender. Fold in soup, water, Worcestershire, pepper, tuna. Cook over moderate heat, stirring constantly, until heated. Serve over rice.

Servings: 4

Exchange per serving: 1½ meat, 1 bread, 1 fruit, 1 fat

# Tasty Tuna

| Ingredients | Measure | Carbohydrates (gm.) | Protein (gm.) | Fat (gm. |
|---|---|---|---|---|
| Cream of mushroom soup | 1 10¾-ounce can | 22.5 | 5.1 | 26. |
| Skim milk | ¼ cup | 3 | 2 | |
| Peas, frozen, cooked and drained | 1 10-ounce package | 36 | 15 | . |
| Tuna, drained and flaked | 1 7-ounce can | | 36.4 | 17. |
| Croutons | ½ cup | 7 | 2 | |
| | | 68.5 | 60.5 | 44. |

Calories: 1 serving—303.9

| | | 22.8 | 20.1 | 14. |
|---|---|---|---|---|

In saucepan blend soup and milk. Add peas and tuna. Heat, stirring occasionally. Garnish with croutons.

Servings: 3
Exchange per serving: 2 meat, 1½ bread, 1 fat

# Tuna Miniatures

| Ingredients | Measure | Carbohydrates (gm.) | Protein (gm.) | Fat (gm.) |
|---|---|---|---|---|
| Crushed corn flakes | 2 cups | 40 | 5 | |
| Milk | ⅓ cup | 4 | 2.5 | 3.3 |
| Mayonnaise | ¼ cup | | | 60 |
| Tuna, drained, water packed | 1 7-ounce can | | 36.4 | 17.2 |
| Parsley | 1 tablespoon | | | |
| Lemon juice | 1 teaspoon | | | |
| Worcestershire sauce | ½ teaspoon | | | |
| Salt | ¼ teaspoon | | | |
| Pepper | dash | | | |
| | | 44 | 43.9 | 80.5 |
| Calories: 1 serving—268.5 | | 11 | 10.9 | 20.1 |

Mix one cup corn flakes with milk and then mix in remaining ingredients. Form one-inch balls. Roll in remaining corn flakes. Bake at 425 degrees on well greased cookie sheet for 15 minutes.

Servings: 4
Exchange per serving: 1½ meat, 1 fruit, 2½ fat

RECIPE FOR

# Tuna-Rice Pie

| Ingredients | Measure | Carbohy-drates (gm.) | Pro-tein (gm.) | Fat (gm.) |
|---|---|---|---|---|
| Instant rice | 1 cup | 60 | 8 | |
| Water | 1 cup | | | |
| Salt | 1 teaspoon | | | |
| Margarine | 1½ teaspoons | | | 7.5 |
| Eggs | 3 | | 21 | 15 |
| American cheese | 1 cup | | 35 | 25 |
| Tuna, drained, water packed | 1 7-ounce can | | 36.4 | 17.2 |
| Milk, skim, scalded | ¾ cup | 9 | 6 | |
| Nutmeg | ⅛ teaspoon | | | |
| Pepper | ⅛ teaspoon | | | |
| | | 69 | 106.4 | 64.7 |

Calories: 1 serving—213.1                 11.5   17.7   10.7

Place rice in 9-inch pie pan. Bring water, ½ teaspoon salt, and margarine to a boil. Stir into rice, cover, let stand 5 minutes. Beat 1 egg slightly, blend into rice. Press against bottom and sides, not above rim, of pie pan. Sprinkle ½ cup cheese on rice crust. Top with half the tuna. Repeat with remaining cheese and then remaining tuna. Blend ½ teaspoon salt, 2 eggs, milk, nutmeg, and pepper. Pour over tuna. Bake at 400 degrees for 25 minutes. If desired, top with tomato wedges for last 5 minutes of baking.

Servings: 6
Exchange per serving: 2 meat, ½ skim milk, ½ fruit

# Seafood Salad

| Ingredients | Measure | Car-bohy-drates (gm.) | Pro-tein (gm.) | Fat (gm.) |
|---|---|---|---|---|
| Crabmeat, tuna, or salmon | 1 cup | | 28 | 20 |
| Lemon juice | ½ teaspoon | | | |
| Onion, finely minced | ½ teaspoon | | | |
| Salt | as desired | | | |
| Paprika | as desired | | | |
| Celery, diced | ½ cup | | | |
| Lettuce hearts, in small pieces | ½ cup | | | |
| Mayonnaise | 4 teaspoons | | | 20 |
| | | | 28 | 40 |
| Calories: 1 serving—236 | | | 14 | 20 |

Lightly mix first seven ingredients in order. Chill thoroughly. Just before serving toss with mayonnaise to moisten. Serve on crisp lettuce.

Servings: 2
Exchange per serving: 2 meat, 2 fat

# Chapter XIII

# Dairy

# Deviled Eggs

| Ingredients | Measure | Carbohydrates (gm.) | Protein (gm.) | Fat (gm.) |
|---|---|---|---|---|
| Eggs, hard cooked | 6 | | 42 | 30 |
| Mayonnaise | ¼ cup | | | 60 |
| Worcestershire sauce | ½ teaspoon | | | |
| Dry mustard | ¼ teaspoon | | | |
| Salt | dash | | | |
| | | | 42 | 90 |
| Calories: 1 serving—163 | | | 7 | 15 |

Remove egg yolks and mash. Blend with remaining ingredients and spoon into egg-white shells.

Servings: 6
Exchange per serving: 1 meat, 2 fat

# Cheese Blintzes

| Ingredients | Measure | Carbohydrates (gm.) | Protein (gm.) | Fat (gm.) |
|---|---|---|---|---|
| Filling: Cottage cheese | ½ pound | | 28 | 20 |
| Egg | 1 | | 7 | 5 |
| Salt | ¼ teaspoon | | | |
| Artificial sweetener | = ¼ teaspoon sugar | | | |
| Cinnamon | ⅛ teaspoon | | | |
| Flour | 1 cup | 75.9 | 10.8 | .◆ |
| Milk, skim | 1 cup | 12 | 8 | |
| Eggs | 4 | | 28 | 20 |
| Salt | ½ teaspoon | | | |
| Margarine, melted | 1 tablespoon | | | 15 |
| Sour cream | 8 tablespoons | | | 20 |
| | | 87.9 | 81.8 | 80.◆ |
| Calories: 1 serving—260.2 | | 21.9 | 20.2 | 10.◆ |

Combine filling and set aside. Sift flour and salt together. Beat eggs; add milk while beating. Gradually add flour. Heat small frying pan. (Teflon is perfect for nonfat cooking here.) Pour ¼ cup batter in pan and tilt to spread thinly. When edges brown and top bubbles, turn out onto clean towel, brown side up. Put 1 tablespoon filling in center and fold up. Place in lightly greased baking dish. Continue with rest of batter and filling. Brush tops with melted margarine and bake at 350 degrees for 30 minutes. Top each blintz with tablespoon sour cream.

Servings: 4 (2 blintzes each)
Exchange per serving: 2 meat, 1 bread, 1 vegetable B, 2 fat

# Cheese Souffle

| Ingredients | Measure | | Carbohydrates (gm.) | Protein (gm.) | Fat (gm.) |
|---|---|---|---|---|---|
| Bisquick | ¼ | cup | 19 | 2.3 | 3.6 |
| Dry mustard | ½ | teaspoon | | | |
| Milk, skim | 1 | cup | 12 | 8 | |
| Grated cheese | 1 | cup | | 35 | 25 |
| Eggs, separated | 3 | | | 21 | 15 |
| Cream of tartar | ¼ | teaspoon | | | |
| | | | 31 | 66.3 | 43.6 |
| Calories: 1 serving—128.8 | | | 5 | 11 | 7.2 |

Mix Bisquick and mustard in saucepan; add small amount of milk to make a paste. Stir in rest of milk gradually. Bring to boil; boil 1 minute, stirring constantly. Stir in cheese. Remove from heat; stir gradually into egg yolks. Beat egg whites and cream of tartar until stiff. Fold in cheese mixture. Pour into ungreased 1½-quart baking dish. Set baking dish in pan of hot water (1 inch deep). Bake at 350 degrees 50 to 60 minutes, or until knife inserted near center comes out clean. Serve with mushroom sauce. (Recipe below.)

Servings: 6
Exchange per serving: 1 meat, ½ skim milk, ½ fat

# Mushroom Sauce

| Ingredients | Measure | | Car-bohy-drates (gm.) | Pro-tein (gm.) | Fat (gm.) |
|---|---|---|---|---|---|
| Egg | 1 | | | 7 | 5 |
| Milk, skim | ½ | cup | 6 | 4 | |
| Lemon juice | 1 | teaspoon | | | |
| Parsley | 1 | teaspoon | | | |
| Onion | 2 | tablespoons | | | |
| Salt | ½ | teaspoon | | | |
| Pepper | | dash | | | |
| Sliced mushrooms, drained | 1 | 4-ounce can | | | |
| | | | 6 | 11 | 5 |
| Calories: 1 serving—27.6 | | | 1.5 | 2.7 | 1.2 |

Put all ingredients into blender. Cover and blend on high speed for 10 seconds. Cook over simmering water in double boiler, stirring occasionally, for 10 minutes.

Servings: 4
Exchange per serving: ¼ meat

# Creole Casserole

| Ingredients | Measure | Car-bohy-drates (gm.) | Pro-tein (gm.) | Fat (gm.) |
|---|---|---|---|---|
| Instant rice | 1 cup | 60 | 8 | |
| Cheddar cheese, grated | 2 cups | | 112 | 80 |
| Tomatoes, with juice | 1 20-ounce can | | | |
| Salt | 1 teaspoon | | | |
| Onion, finely chopped | ¼ cup | 3.5 | 1 | |
| | | 63.5 | 121 | 80 |
| Calories: 1 serving—363.2 | | 15.8 | 30 | 20 |

Spread ½ cup rice, right from the box, in a layer on bottom of greased 1½-quart baking dish. Cover with 1 cup of the cheese. Add remaining rice. Combine tomatoes and juice, salt, and onion in saucepan, crushing tomatoes and mixing well. Bring to boil. Pour over layers of rice and cheese. Bake, covered, at 350 degrees for 10 minutes. Remove from oven, uncover, spoon remaining cheese around edge of rice mixture, leaving center uncovered. Bake 5 minutes longer.

Servings: 4
Exchange per serving: 4 meat, 1 bread

# Baked Eggs

| Ingredients | Measure | | Carbohydrates (gm.) | Protein (gm.) | Fat (gm.) |
|---|---|---|---|---|---|
| Egg | 1 | | | 7 | 5 |
| Milk, skim | 2 | tablespoons | 1.5 | 1 | |
| Salt | | as desired | | | |
| Pepper | | as desired | | | |
| Calories: 1 serving—83 | | | 1.5 | 8 | 5 |

Butter small custard cup lightly; spoon milk into cup. Break egg in cup sprinkle with salt and pepper. Bake at 325 degrees for 20 minutes or until eggs are cooked as you like them. Serve in cups.

Servings: 1
Exchange per serving: 1 meat, ⅛ skim milk

# Omelet

| Ingredients | Measure | Carbohydrates (gm.) | Protein (gm.) | Fat (gm.) |
|---|---|---|---|---|
| Eggs, separated | 4 | | 28 | 20 |
| Hot water | 4 tablespoons | | | |
| Salt | as desired | | | |
| Pepper | as desired | | | |
| | | | 28 | 20 |
| Calories: 1 serving—146 | | | 14 | 10 |

Beat yolks till thick and creamy. Add water and seasonings. Beat egg whites until stiff but not dry and fold into yolks. Pour egg mixture into heated pan (Teflon is perfect for nonfat cooking here) and cook over low heat until brown on bottom and dry on top (Insert knife in center; if it comes out dry, omelet is done.) Fold over and turn on a heated platter.

You can insert any of the following fillings in center of omelet before folding over:

1. 3 spears cooked asparagus—free
2. ½ ounce grated cheese—½ meat exchange
3. 2 teaspoons dietetic jam or jelly—free
4. ½ ounce sauteed cubes of sausage—½ meat, ½ fat exchange
5. ½ ounce cooked meat or chicken—½ meat exchange

Servings: 2
Exchange per serving: 2 meat

# CHAPTER XIV

# Fats

## FAT

| Fat      | 5  |
|----------|----|
| Calories | 45 |

| | |
|---|---|
| Butter or margarine | 1 teaspoon |
| Bacon, crisp | 1 slice |
| Cream, light 20 percent | 2 tablespoons |
| Cream, heavy 40 percent | 1 tablespoon |
| Cream cheese | 1 tablespoon |
| French dressing | 1 tablespoon |
| Mayonnaise | 1 teaspoon |
| Oil or cooking fat | 1 teaspoon |
| Chopped walnuts | 1 tablespoon |
| Olives | 5 small |
| Avocado | ⅛ (4-inch diameter) |
| Sour cream | 2 tablespoons |

Nuts:

| | |
|---|---|
| Almonds | 10 |
| Cashews | 5 |
| Peanuts | 10 |
| Pecans | 7 |
| Brazil | 2 |
| Pistachio | 20 |
| Black walnuts | 5 halves or 1 tablespoon |
| English walnuts, chopped | 1 tablespoon |
| Filberts | 5 |

The new Teflon pans make it possible to cook many foods without using any fat at all.

The new whipped margarine is calculated exactly the same as regular stick margarine. However, because of its consistency, you will find that one teaspoon of the whipped will go much farther than one teaspoon of the stick.

# Chapter XV

# Soups and Lunches

CAMPBELL'S SOUPS

Exchange substitutions for 1 bread and ½ fat:
        Frozen green pea with ham
        Green pea

Exchange substitution for 1 bread:
        Black bean
        Tomato
        Tomato rice
        Vegetable
        Vegetable bean

Exchange substitutions for ½ bread and ½ fat:
        Asparagus, cream of
        Beef noodle
        Chicken gumbo
        Chicken noodle
        Potato, cream of
        Turkey noodle
        Turkey vegetable
        Vegetarian vegetable

Exchange substitutions for ½ meat and ½ bread:
        Beef soup
        Chicken vegetable
        Clam chowder, Manhattan style
        Pepper pot
        Scotch broth
        Vegetable beef
        Frozen vegetable with beef, old-fashioned

Exchange substitutions for ½ bread and 1 fat:
        Celery, cream of
        Chicken, cream of

Minestrone
Frozen potato, cream of
Vegetable, cream of

Exchange substitution for 1 meat and 1 bread:
Split pea with ham

Products that may be served without measuring:
Beef broth
Consomme
Tomato juice
V-8 Cocktail vegetable juice

These recommendations are based on a 100-gram portion, which is equiva
lent to 3½ ounces or ⅓ can soup. This makes a 7-ounce serving when pre
pared according to the directions on the label.

## OTHER CAMPBELL'S PRODUCTS IN EXCHANGE LISTS

Exchange substitutions for 1 bread:
Red Kettle vegetable dry soup mix
Red Kettle cream of potato dry soup mix (use milk listed in your
diet)

Exchange substitutions for ½ bread and ½ fat:
Red Kettle cream of mushroom dry soup mix (use milk listed in
your diet)
Red Kettle noodle dry soup mix (based on 4 8-ounce servings per
can)
Red Kettle onion dry soup mix

Exchange substitutions for 1 meat and ½ bread:
Bounty chili con carne (½ cup)

Exchange substitutions for ½ meat and 1 vegetable B:
Bounty beef stew (½ cup)
Bounty chicken stew (½ cup)

Exchange substitutions for ½ meat and ½ bread:
Red Kettle chicken noodle dry soup mix
Red Kettle beef noodle dry soup mix
Red Kettle old-fashioned beef dry soup mix

(All soup mixes based on 3 8-ounce servings per can unless otherwise noted.)

## HEINZ PRODUCTS IN DIABETIC EXCHANGE LISTS:

One cup of soup means ½ cup soup as taken from the can plus ½ cup water. If desired, ½ cup milk taken from the daily allotment may be used in place of the water.

SOUPS (1 cup each):

| | |
|---|---|
| Alphabet with vegetables | ½ bread, 1 fat |
| Bean, with smoked pork | 1½ bread, 1 meat |
| Beef noodle | ½ bread, ½ fat |
| Beef, vegetable and barley | ½ bread, ½ meat |
| Celery, cream of | ½ bread, 1 fat |
| Chicken, cream of | ½ bread, 1 fat |
| Chicken gumbo | ½ bread, ½ fat |
| Chicken noodle | ½ bread, ½ fat |
| Chicken vegetable | ½ bread, ½ meat |
| Chicken with rice | ½ bread, ½ fat |
| Chili with beef | 1 bread, 1 meat, ½ fat |
| Clam chowder (Manhattan style) | ½ bread, ½ fat |
| Consomme (chicken) | free |
| Green pea, cream of | 1½ bread, ½ fat |
| Minestrone | 1 bread, ½ fat |
| Mushroom, cream of | 2 fat, ½ bread |
| Split pea | 1½ bread, 1 meat |
| Tomato | 1 bread, ½ fat |
| Tomato with rice | 1 bread, 1 fat |
| Turkey noodle | ½ bread, ½ fat |
| Turtle, genuine | ½ bread |
| Vegetable beef | 1 bread, ½ fat |
| Vegetable with beef broth | 1 bread, ½ fat |
| Vegetable without meat | 1 bread, ½ fat |

MINUTE MEALS:

| | |
|---|---|
| Beef stew (1 cup) | 1 bread, 2 meat |
| Chicken noodle dinner (1 cup) | 1 bread, 1 meat |

Chicken stew with dumplings
(1 cup)                                       1 bread, 2 fat
Macaroni with cheese sauce (1 cup)   1½ bread, 1 meat, 1 fat
Macaroni creole (¾ cup)               1½ bread, ½ fat

## BEANS (½ cup):

With pork and molasses sauce          1 meat, 2 bread
With pork and tomato sauce            1 meat, 1½ bread

## LIPTON SOUP:

1 serving onion (4 per package)       ½ bread
1 serving cream of mushroom           ½ bread
(4 per package)

## CHEF BOY-AR-DEE:

Ravioli with beef (1⅝-ounce can)      2½ bread, 1 fat
Spaghetti and meatballs
(1⅝-ounce can)                        2 bread, 1 meat, ½ fat
Pizza pie mix (with water) (¼ total)  2 bread, 1 fat
Spaghetti and meatball dinner
(1/6 total)                           3 bread, 1 meat
Spaghetti with meat dinner
(1/6 total)                           2½ bread, 1 meat
Spaghetti with mushroom dinner
(1/6 total)                           2½ bread
Pizza with sausage (1/6 total)        1½ bread, ½ meat, 1 fat
Frozen beef ravioli (8-ounces)
(½ can)                               2½ bread, 1 meat, 1 fat
Frozen cheese ravioli (8-ounces)
(½ can)                               2 bread, 1 meat, 1 fat
Beefaroni 5-ounces (⅓ can)            1 bread, 1 meat
Ravioli 5-ounces (⅓ can)              1½ bread, ½ meat, 1 fat
Chili con carne with beans
(5-ounces) (⅓ can)                    1½ bread, 1 fat
Meat balls with gravy (5-ounces)
(⅓ can)                               ½ bread, 2 meat, 1 fat

| | |
|---|---|
| Ravioli with beef (5-ounces) (⅓ can) | 1½ bread, 1 fat |
| Spaghetti and meatballs (5-ounces) (⅓ can) | 1 bread, 1 meat |
| Meatball stew (7-ounces) (¼ can) | 1 bread, 1 meat, 1 fat |
| Lasagna (8-ounces) (1/5 can) | 2 bread, 1 meat, 1 fat |
| Frozen lasagna (8-ounces) (½ can) | 1½ bread, 2 meat, 1 fat |
| Frozen manicotti (8-ounces) (½ can) | 2 bread, 2 meat, 3 fat |

CHUN KING CHINESE FOOD:

| | |
|---|---|
| Chow mein chicken divider pack (¼ total) | 2 bread, 2 meat |
| Chow mein beef divider pack (¼ total) | 2 bread, 2 meat, 1 fat |
| Chow mein mushroom divider pack (¼ total) | 2 bread |
| Chow mein meatless divider pack (½ can) | 1 bread |
| Subgum chicken chow mein (½ can) | 1 bread |
| Beef chop suey (½ can) | 1 bread |
| Chinese vegetables (½ can) | free |
| Chop suey vegetables (½ can) | free |
| Bean sprouts (½ can) | free |
| Chow mein noodles (½ can) | 1½ bread, 2 fat |
| Frozen chicken chow mein (8-ounces) (½ package) | 1 bread, 1 meat |
| Soy sauce | free |

# Quiche Lorraine

| Ingredients | Measure | | Carbohydrates (gm.) | Protein (gm.) | Fat (gm.) |
|---|---|---|---|---|---|
| Swiss cheese, shredded | 8 | ounces | | 56 | 40 |
| Eggs | 3 | | | 21 | 15 |
| Milk, skim | 1½ | cups | 18 | 12 | |
| Salt | ¾ | teaspoon | | | |
| Pepper | | dash | | | |
| Onion flakes | 2 | tablespoons | | | |
| Margarine | 1 | tablespoon | | | 15 |
| 9-inch pie shell | 1 | | 96 | 14 | 81 |
| | | | 114 | 103 | 151 |
| Calories: 1 serving—369 | | | 19 | 17 | 25 |

Spread cheese and onion flakes in bottom of pie shell. Beat milk, eggs, salt, and pepper in a bowl to blend. Pour into shell. Dot with margarine. Bake 375 degrees for 40 minutes. Allow to stand 10 minutes.

Servings: 6
Exchange per serving: 2 meat, 1½ bread, 3 fat

# Chilled Pea Soup

| Ingredients | Measure | Carbohydrates (gm.) | Protein (gm.) | Fat (gm.) |
|---|---|---|---|---|
| Frozen peas | 20 ounces | 35 | 10 | |
| Artificial sweetener | = 2 teaspoons sugar | | | |
| Onion, cut up | ½ | | | |
| Margarine | 3 tablespoons | | | 45 |
| Flour | 3 tablespoons | 33.6 | 3 | |
| Salt | 2 teaspoons | | | |
| Pepper | dash | | | |
| Milk, skim | 3 cups | 36 | 24 | |
| Water | 2 cups | | | |
| Egg white, hard cooked, chopped | 1 | .2 | 3.3 | |
| | | 104.8 | 40.3 | 45 |
| Calories: 1 serving—211.6 | | 17.7 | 10 | 11.2 |

Day before or early in the day, cook peas with salt, according to label. Drain, place in blender with onion; cover; blend smooth on high speed. In saucepan melt margarine; stir in flour, salt, and pepper; slowly stir in milk; then cook, stirring, until slightly thickened. Remove from heat and stir in pea mixture and water. Refrigerate. Serve cold, garnished with chopped, hard cooked egg white.

Servings: 6
Exchange per serving: 1 bread, 1 meat, 1 fat

# Chilled Tomato Creme Soup

| Ingredients | Measure | Carbohydrates (gm.) | Protein (gm.) | Fat (gm.) |
|---|---|---|---|---|
| Frozen cream of potato soup | ½ of a 10¾-ounce can | 15 | 4 | 6.4 |
| Tabasco | dash | | | |
| Seasoned salt | 2 teaspoons | | | |
| Horse radish | 2 teaspoons | | | |
| Tomato, large, quartered | 1 | | | |
| Canned tomato juice | 1½ cups | | | |
| Croutons | 1 slice bread | 15 | 2 | |
| | | 30 | 6 | 6.4 |
| Calories: 1 serving—50.4 | | 7.5 | 1.5 | 1.6 |

Early in day combine all ingredients, except tomato juice and crouton, in blender. Cover, blend smooth on high speed. Add tomato juice, cover, blend 1 minute. Refrigerate. Stir soup well, pour into glasses. Top with few croutons.

Servings: 4
Exchange per serving: 1 vegetable B

# Tomato Bouillon

| Ingredients | Measure | Car-bohy-drates (gm.) | Pro-tein (gm.) | Fat (gm.) |
|---|---|---|---|---|
| Beef bouillon | 2 cans | | | |
| Tomato soup | 2 cans | 73.8 | 8.4 | 9.6 |
| Basil | dash | | | |
| Water | 3 soup cans | | | |
| | | 73.8 | 8.4 | 9.6 |
| Calories: 1 serving—40.5 | | 7.3 | .8 | .9 |

Combine all ingredients; simmer a few minutes.

Servings: 10
Exchange per serving: ⅔ fruit

# Egg Drop Soup

| Ingredients | Measure | Carbohydrates (gm.) | Protein (gm.) | Fat (gm. |
|---|---|---|---|---|
| Condensed beef broth | 1 10½-ounce can | | | |
| Water | 2 soup cans | | | |
| Bay leaf | ½ medium | | | |
| Egg | 1 | | 7 | 5 |
| | | | 7 | 5 |

Calories: 1 serving—                                              1.1      .8

Combine soup, water, and bay leaf. Bring to a boil. Beat egg slightly slowly pour it in a thin stream into soup, stirring constantly. Remove bay leaf. Egg should form thin threads.

Servings: 6
Exchange per serving: free

# Chicken Soup

| Ingredients | Measure | Carbohydrates (gm.) | Protein (gm.) | Fat (gm.) |
|---|---|---|---|---|
| Chicken, stewing | 3 pounds (including bone) | | | |
| Salt | 4 teaspoons | | | |
| Water | 3 quarts | | | |
| Celery | 3 cups | | | |
| Onion, quartered | 3 | | | |
| Carrots | 3 cups | | | |
| Pepper | 6 cloves | | | |

Combine all ingredients in a large pot; bring to a boil and simmer, covered, 4 hours. Remove chicken (can be used for chicken salad or chicken chow mein). Pour soup through strainer (reserve vegetables) and let stand so fat will rise to top; skim off fat.

Place ¼ cup cooked noodles in bowl; add ¼ cup cooked vegetables from soup; pour in ½ cup soup; top with knaidlach (recipe below).

Servings: 15
Exchange per serving: 1 bread, 1 fat, 1 vegetable B (½ bread for noodles, ½ bread for knaidlach, vegetable B for vegetables)

# Airy Knaidlach (Dumplings for Chicken Soup)

| Ingredients | Measure | | Carbohydrates (gm.) | Protein (gm.) | Fat (gm.) |
|---|---|---|---|---|---|
| Eggs | 4 | | | 28 | 20 |
| Matzo meal | 1 | cup | 120 | 16 | |
| Salt | 1½ | teaspoons | | | |
| Oil | 4 | tablespoons | | | 60 |
| Water | 2 | tablespoons | | | |
| | | | 120 | 44 | 80 |

Calories: 1 serving—85.8      7.5   2.7   5

Early in day mix oil and eggs together. Add matzo meal and salt. Then add water. Refrigerate. 40 minutes before serving bring 3 quarts water to boil. Reduce flame so water bubbles slightly and drop in balls of mixture. Cover pot and cook 40 minutes.

Servings: 16
Exchange per serving: ½ bread, 1 fat

# Pizza on English Muffins

| Ingredients | Measure | | Carbohydrates (gm.) | Protein (gm.) | Fat (gm.) |
|---|---|---|---|---|---|
| Onion, chopped | ¼ | cup | 3.5 | 1 | |
| Olive or salad oil | 2 | tablespoons | | | 30 |
| Tomatoes | 1 | 19-ounce can | | | |
| Bay leaf | 1 | | | | |
| Salt | 1 | teaspoon | | | |
| Artificial sweetener | = 1 | teaspoon sugar | | | |
| Oregano | ½ | teaspoon | | | |
| Pepper | | dash | | | |
| English muffins | 4 | | 60 | 8 | 10 |
| Mozzarella cheese | 4 | 1-ounce slices | | 28 | 20 |
| | | | 63.5 | 37 | 60 |
| Calories: 1 pizza—117 | | | 7.9 | 4.6 | 7.5 |

Brown onion in oil. Add remaining ingredients, except for muffins and cheese, cover, and cook slowly for 30 minutes. Stir occasionally. Split English muffins in half and place cut side up on cookie sheet. Spoon sauce on each side; top each pizza with ½ slice cheese. Bake at 450 degrees for 12 minutes.

Servings: 4 (2 pizzas per serving)

Exchange per serving: 1 bread, 1 meat, 2 fat

# Shrimp Toast

| Ingredients | Measure | Carbohydrates (gm.) | Protein (gm.) | Fat (gm.) |
|---|---|---|---|---|
| Frozen shrimp, thawed | 10 medium | | 14 | 10 |
| Bread | 2 slices | 30 | 4 | |
| Mayonnaise | ¼ cup | | | 30 |
| American cheese, diced | 2 1-ounce slices | | 14 | 10 |
| Curry powder | dash | | | |
| | | 30 | 32 | 50 |
| Calories: 1 serving—349 | | 15 | 16 | 25 |

Cut bread in half, diagonally and place on broiler pan. Place shrimp on bread in single layer. Mix mayonnaise, cheese and curry powder and spread over shrimp. Broil 1-2 minutes 3-4 inches from heat or until topping starts to brown. Serve at once.

Servings: 2
Exchange per serving: 2 meat, 1 bread, 3 fat

# CHAPTER XVI

# Sauces and Toppings

DREAM WHIP (free, in ordinary amounts)

1 tablespoon
Carbohydrate .6 gm.
Protein .3 gm.
Fat .6 gm.

FRENCH'S SAUCE AND GRAVY MIXES—
4 SERVINGS PER PACKAGE

|  | 1 serving |
|---|---|
| Beef stew seasoning | ¼ bread |
| Brown gravy | ⅛ bread |
| Cheese sauce | ⅛ bread |
| Chicken gravy | ¼ bread |
| Chili-O | ½ bread |
| Hollandaise sauce | ⅛ bread |
| Mushroom gravy | ⅛ bread |
| Newburg sauce | ¼ bread |
| Onion gravy | ¼ bread |
| Sloppy joe | ½ bread |
| Sour cream sauce | ⅛ bread |
| Spaghetti sauce (Italian) | ½ bread |
| Spaghetti sauce with mushrooms | ¼ bread |
| Stroganoff | ½ bread |

# Tangy Cocktail Sauce

| Ingredients | Measure | | Car-bohy-drates (gm.) | Pro-tein (gm.) | Fat (gm.) |
|---|---|---|---|---|---|
| Catsup | ½ cup | | 39.2 | 3.2 | |
| Parsley | 1 teaspoon | | | | |
| Horse radish | 1 teaspoon | | | | |
| Lemon juice | 1 teaspoon | | | | |
| Salt | ½ teaspoon | | | | |
| Worcestershire sauce | ½ teaspoon | | | | |
| Artificial sweetener | = | 2 teaspoons sugar | | | |
| | | | 39.2 | 3.2 | |
| Calories: 2 tablespoons—42.4 | | | 9.8 | .8 | |

Blend ingredients well. Chill to blend flavors. Excellent served as a dip for raw cauliflower.

Servings: Yield—½ cup
Exchange per serving: 2 tablespoons=1 fruit

# Hot Barbecue Sauce

| Ingredients | Measure | Carbohydrates (gm.) | Protein (gm.) | Fat (gm.) |
|---|---|---|---|---|
| Lemon juice | ½ cup | | | |
| Tomato juice | ¼ cup | | | |
| Salt | 1 teaspoon | | | |
| Paprika | 1 teaspoon | | | |
| Pepper | ½ teaspoon | | | |
| Onion powder | ½ teaspoon | | | |
| Margarine | 1 teaspoon | | | 5 |
| Cider vinegar | ⅓ cup | | | |
| Cold water | ¼ cup | | | |
| Dry mustard | 1 teaspoon | | | |
| Artificial sweetener | = 2½ teaspoons sugar | | | |
| Red pepper | ½ teaspoon | | | |
| Tabasco sauce | 1 teaspoon | | | |
| Garlic powder | ⅛ teaspoon | | | |

Combine ingredients in saucepan and heat to boiling point.

Servings: 1½ cups

Exchange per serving: free

# Polynesian Barbecue Sauce

| Ingredients | Measure | Carbohydrates (gm.) | Protein (gm.) | Fat (gm. |
|---|---|---|---|---|
| Tomato juice | 1½ cups | | | |
| Soy sauce | ½ cup | | | |
| Garlic, crushed | 3 cloves | | | |
| Worcestershire sauce | 1 tablespoon | | | |
| Hot pepper sauce | few drops | | | |
| Lemon juice | 1 lemon | | | |

Combine all ingredients.

Servings: 2 cups
Exchange per serving: free

# Seafood Sauce

| Ingredients | Measure | Carbohydrates (gm.) | Protein (gm.) | Fat (gm.) |
|---|---|---|---|---|
| Mayonnaise | ¼ cup | | | 30 |
| Catsup | ¼ cup | 19.6 | 1.2 | |
| Parsley, minced | 1 tablespoon | | | |
| Horseradish | 1 teaspoon | | | |
| Onion, grated | 1 teaspoon | | | |
| | | 19.6 | 1.2 | 30 |
| Calories: 1 tablespoon—43.3 | | 2.4 | .1 | 3.7 |

Combine all ingredients, stirring until well blended. Serve over broiled fish fillet.

Servings: 8 tablespoons
Exchange per serving: 1 tablespoon—1 fat

159

# Ruby Strawberry Sauce

| Ingredients | Measure | Carbohydrates (gm.) | Protein (gm.) | Fat (gm.) |
|---|---|---|---|---|
| Strawberries, washed and hulled | 1 pint | 20 | | |
| Artificial sweetener | = 32 teaspoons sugar | | | |
| Cornstarch | 2 tablespoons | 15 | 2 | |
| Water | ½ cup | | | |
| | | 35 | 2 | |
| Calories: 1 serving—18 | | 4.3 | .2 | |

Slice half of strawberries and set aside. Mash other half in small bowl. Mix artificial sweetener and cornstarch in medium saucepan; stir in water and mashed strawberries. Cook, stirring constantly, until mixture thickens and boils 3 minutes. Strain into medium-size bowl; fold in sliced strawberries.

Serve warm or cold over ice cream, vanilla pudding, or slices of angel cake or pound cake.

Servings: 8
Exchange per serving: ½ fruit

# Gelatin Whipped Cream

| Ingredients | Measure | Car-bohy-drates (gm.) | Pro-tein (gm.) | Fat (gm.) |
|---|---|---|---|---|
| Dietetic gelatin, any flavor | 1 envelope | | | |
| Hot water | ½ cup | | | |
| Light cream | 1 cup | | | 40 |
| | | | | 40 |

Calories: 1 serving—45      5

Dissolve gelatin in hot water. Chill until slightly thickened. Add cream and beat until light and fluffy (about 1 minute). Chill several minutes to set lightly. Before using, stir until smooth and fluffy, like whipped cream. Serve on gelatin, cake, or pudding.

Servings: 2 cups
Exchange per serving: ¼ cup=1 fat

# Whipped Topping

| Ingredients | Measure | | Carbohydrates (gm.) | Protein (gm.) | Fat (gm. |
|---|---|---|---|---|---|
| Nonfat dry milk solids | ¼ cup | | 12 | 8 | |
| Ice water | ¼ cup | | | | |
| Artificial sweetener | = | 4 teaspoons sugar | | | |
| | | | 12 | 8 | |
| Calories: 1 serving—20 | | | 3 | 2 | |

Combine ingredients and beat on high speed of mixer until of consistenc of whipped cream.

Servings: 4
Exchange per serving: ¼ skimmed milk

# Pretend Sour Cream

| Ingredients | Measure | Carbohydrates (gm.) | Protein (gm.) | Fat (gm.) |
|---|---|---|---|---|
| Lemon juice | 2 tablespoons | | | |
| Milk, skim | ¼ cup | 3 | 2 | |
| Cottage cheese | 1 cup | | 28 | 20 |
| Salt | pinch | | | |
| | | 3 | 30 | 20 |
| Calories: 2 tablespoons—40.1 | | .7 | 3.7 | 2.5 |

Place lemon juice and milk in blender. Gradually add cottage cheese and salt, blending at low speed. Blend a few minutes at high speed until smooth. If mixture thickens on standing, thin with additional milk but be sure to calculate the addition.

Servings: 1 cup
Exchange per serving: 2 tablespoons=½ meat

# Chocolate Frosting

| Ingredients | Measure | Carbohy-drates (gm.) | Pro-tein (gm.) | Fat (gm.) |
|---|---|---|---|---|
| Unsweetened chocolate | 1 ounce | 8 | 4 | 15.1 |
| Evaporated milk | 6 tablespoons | 9 | 6 | 7.5 |
| Vanilla | ½ teaspoon | | | |
| Artificial sweetener | = 8 teaspoons sugar | | | |
| | | 17 | 10 | 22.6 |
| Calories: 1 serving—39.6 | | 2.1 | 1.5 | 2.8 |

Melt chocolate over hot water. Stir in milk. Mix well and cook until thickened, about 2 or 3 minutes. Remove from heat and stir in vanilla and artificial sweetener. If too thick, thin down with water.

Servings: 8
Exchange per serving: ½ fat, 1/6 skim milk

# Cream Cheese Frosting

| Ingredients | Measure | Carbohydrates (gm.) | Protein (gm.) | Fat (gm.) |
|---|---|---|---|---|
| Cream cheese | 4 tablespoons | | | 20 |
| Dietetic pineapple or strawberry jam | 2 teaspoons | | | |
| | | | | 20 |

Calories: 1 serving—45      5

Soften cream cheese at room temperature for 30 minutes. Add jam spread and beat vigorously with mixer. Spread on cake or cupcakes, allowing 1 tablespoon per serving.

Variations: To plain cream cheese add:

1. 1 tablespoon milk and artificial sweetener—1 teaspoon sugar, 2 drops vanilla
2. Few drops artificial coloring
3. ¼ teaspoon grated orange rind
4. ⅛ to ¼ teaspoon grated lemon rind

Servings: 4
Exchange per serving: 1 fat

# Cheese and Mushroom Ball

| Ingredients | Measure | Carbohydrates (gm.) | Protein (gm.) | Fat (gm.) |
|---|---|---|---|---|
| Mushrooms, sliced, drained | 1  4½-ounce can | | | |
| Cream cheese, softened | 8-ounces | | | 80 |
| Onion, finely minced | 1  tablespoon | | | |
| Salt | ½  teaspoon | | | |
| Worcestershire sauce | 1  teaspoon | | | |
| | | | | 80 |

Calories: 1 teaspoon—14.4                                                    1.6

Chop mushrooms. Mix into cream cheese with onion, salt, and Worcestershire sauce. Chill thoroughly. Shape into ball. Serve with assorted crackers.

Servings: 1 5-inch ball
Exchange per serving: 1 teaspoon—⅓ fat exchange

# Desserts

Recipes calling for one envelope dietetic gelatin or pudding are based on envelopes yielding 2 ½-cup servings. (They would be made by using 1 cup of water or milk.)

If the envelope you use yields 4 ½-cup servings (made by using 2 cups of water or milk) use only one half the contents of the envelope.

Remember that dietetic gelatin can be used in place of regular gelatin and this opens up a wonderful area of light and low calorie desserts. The companies manufacturing regular gelatin often have recipes in magazine advertisements and some offer small cookbooks utilizing their products. By substituting dietetic gelatin in these recipes you will have endless sources of dessert dishes. (Just be sure to calculate the additional ingredients that may be added and deduct them from your meal allowance.)

JOHNSTON GRAHAM CRACKER
AND CHOCOLATE READY-CRUSTS:

⅛ crust—1 bread, 1 fat

# Apple Torte

| Ingredients | Measure | | Carbohydrates (gm.) | Protein (gm.) | Fat (gm.) |
|---|---|---|---|---|---|
| Apples | 8 | | 80 | | |
| Artificial sweetener | = | 1 cup sugar | | | |
| Cinnamon | | as desired | | | |
| Brown sugar | 1 cup | | 240 | | |
| All-purpose flour | 1 cup | | 76 | 11 | .9 |
| Butter or margarine melted | ¼ cup | | | | 60 |
| Pecans, chopped | ½ cup | | | | 40 |
| Cool Whip | | | | | |
| | | | 395 | 11 | 100.9 |

Calories: 1 serving—317      49.3   1.5   12.7

Peel and slice apples. Place in pan 2 inches deep, almost filled with apples (pack down tightly). Sprinkle with ¾ cup artificial sweetener and cinnamon to taste.

Topping: Combine brown sugar, flour, and butter or margarine until crumbly. Place on top of apples, pressing down to form a crust. Sprinkle with pecans. Bake at 375 degrees for 35 minutes or until apples are tender and crust is firm.

Servings: 8
Exchange per serving: 5 fruit, 2½ fat

# Graham Cracker Crust—8 or 9 inch

| Ingredients | Measure | | Carbohydrates (gm.) | Protein (gm.) | Fat (gm.) |
|---|---|---|---|---|---|
| Graham crackers, crushed | 1 cup (12 square) | | 90 | 12 | |
| Margarine, melted | 2 tablespoons | | | | 30 |
| Artificial sweetener | = | 6 teaspoons sugar | | | |
| | | | 90 | 12 | 30 |
| Calories: ⅛ crust—83.7 | | | 11.1 | 1.5 | 3.7 |

Combine ingredients and press into 8- or 9-inch pan. Refrigerate 1 hour before filling.

Servings: 8- or 9-inch crust
Exchange per serving: ⅛ crust=1 fruit, 1 fat

# Rice Crisp Cereal Crust—8 inch

| Ingredients | Measure | | Car-bohy-drates (gm.) | Pro-tein (gm.) | Fat (gm. |
|---|---|---|---|---|---|
| Rice crispy cereal, crushed | 1 cup | | 20 | 2.6 | |
| Margarine, melted | 2 tablespoons | | | | 30 |
| Artificial sweetener | = | 2 teaspoons sugar | | | |
| | | | 20 | 2.6 | 30 |
| Calories: ⅛ crust—44.5 | | | 2.5 | .3 | 3. |

Combine ingredients and press into bottom of 8-inch pie pan. Chill while preparing filling.

Servings: 8-inch crust
Exchange per serving: ⅛ = ¼ fruit, 1 fat

# Pastry (yields 14 tarts or 1 9-inch pie crust)

| Ingredients | Measure | Carbohydrates (gm.) | Protein (gm.) | Fat (gm.) |
|---|---|---|---|---|
| Water | ¼ cup | | | |
| Flour | 1¼ cups | 94.8 | 13.5 | 1.1 |
| Salt | ½ teaspoon | | | |
| Margarine | ¼ pound | | | 120 |
| | | 94.8 | 13.5 | 121.1 |
| Calories: 1 serving—137.7 | | 6.7 | .9 | 8.6 |

Measure water, flour, and salt into small electric mixing bowl. Slice in margarine. Mix on low speed for 20 seconds. Shape into ball and roll out.

Tarts—cut into 14 circles and fit into tart molds. Prick with fork. Bake at 450 for 10 minutes. Fill as desired.

Baked pie shell—fit into 9-inch pie pan. Prick with fork. Bake at 450 for 10 minutes. Fill as desired.

Unbaked pie shell—fit into 9-inch pie pan. Fill as desired and bake according to filling directions.

Servings: 14

Exchange per serving: ½ bread, 1½ fat (Be sure to calculate filling.)

# Cool La La Lime Pie-Filling

| Ingredients | Measure | | Carbohydrates (gm.) | Protein (gm.) | Fat (gm.) |
|---|---|---|---|---|---|
| Eggs | 2 | | | 14 | 10 |
| Artificial sweetener | = ½ cup sugar | | | | |
| Green coloring | few drops | | | | |
| Light cream | 1 cup | | | 7.2 | 40 |
| Lime juice | ⅓ cup | | | | |
| Lime peel | 1 teaspoon | | | | |
| Vanilla ice cream | 1 pint | | 60 | 8 | 40 |
| | | | 60 | 29.2 | 90 |

Calories: 1 serving—157.2   8.7   3.6   11

Beat eggs until thick and lemon colored. Slowly add artificial sweetener and continue beating until mixture is light and fluffy. Add green coloring, cream, lime juice, and grated peel. Mix well. Pour into freezing tray and freeze until firm. Whip vanilla ice cream until smooth and spread into crust. Turn lime mixture into bowl and beat smooth. Pour over ice cream. Freeze.

Servings: 8

Exchange per serving: 1 fruit, ½ meat, 1½ fat (Filling alone—add exchanges for crust you choose to make.)

172

# Cherry Cream Pie Filling

| Ingredients | Measure | Carbohydrates (gm.) | Protein (gm.) | Fat (gm.) |
|---|---|---|---|---|
| Unflavored gelatin | 1 teaspoon | | 7 | |
| Milk, skim | 1 cup | | | |
| | & 2 tablespoons | 13.5 | 9 | |
| Egg, well beaten | 1 | | 7 | 5 |
| Artificial sweetener | = 6 teaspoons sugar | | | |
| Salt | ⅛ teaspoon | | | |
| Vanilla | ½ teaspoon | | | |
| Sour pie cherries | 1 1-pound can | 60 | 4 | 1.6 |
| Cherry juice | ⅔ cup | | | |
| Cornstarch | 2 tablespoons | 15 | 2 | |
| Artificial sweetener | = ¼ cup sugar | | | |
| Almond extract | ⅛ teaspoon | | | |
| Red food coloring | few drops | | | |
| | | 88.5 | 29 | 6.6 |
| Calories: 1 serving—65.6 | | 11 | 3.6 | .8 |

Soften gelatin in 2 tablespoons milk. In double boiler combine egg, 1 cup milk, artificial sweetener (=6 teaspoons sugar), and salt. Cook over boiling water, stirring constantly, until mixture coats a metal spoon. Add vanilla and softened gelatin. Chill until thickened but not set. Drain sour pie cherries, reserving ⅔ cup juice. Combine cornstarch, artificial sweetener (=¼ cup sugar), and cherry juice in saucepan. Blend well. Add cherries; cook over medium heat, stirring constantly, until mixture thickens. Remove from heat. Add almond extract and food coloring. Chill. Turn into crust. Spoon custard over cherries. Chill until firm, 4 to 6 hours.

Servings: 8

Exchange per serving: ½ skim milk, ½ fruit (Filling alone—add exchanges for crust you choose to make.)

# Gelatin Cheese Torte Pie Filling

| Ingredients | Measure | Car-bohy-drates (gm.) | Pro-tein (gm.) | Fat (gm. |
|---|---|---|---|---|
| Dietetic gelatin, any flavor | 1 envelope | | | |
| Boiling water | ½ cup | | | |
| Cream cheese | 4 ounces | | | 40 |
| Artificial sweetener | = ¼ cup sugar | | | |
| Evaporated milk, whipped | ⅔ cup | 16 | 10.6 | 13. |
| | | 16 | 10.6 | 53. |
| Calories: 1 serving—72.6 | | 2 | 1.3 | 6. |

Dissolve gelatin in boiling water. Cool until it just begins to set. Crear together cheese and artificial sweetener. Add gelatin. Mix well. Whip mil according to package directions. Fold whipped milk into gelatin mixture Pour filling into crust. Chill several hours or overnight.

Servings: 8
Exchange per serving: 1/6 milk, 1 fat (Filling alone—add exchanges fo crust you choose to make.)

# Chocolate Bavarian

| Ingredients | Measure | Carbohydrates (gm.) | Protein (gm.) | Fat (gm.) |
|---|---|---|---|---|
| Unflavored gelatin | 1 envelope | | 7 | |
| Water | 2 tablespoons | | | |
| Cocoa | ¼ cup | 14.4 | 2.4 | 6.4 |
| Milk, skim | 1 cup | 12 | 8 | |
| Artificial sweetener | = 16 teaspoons sugar | | | |
| Vanilla | ½ teaspoon | | | |
| Nonfat dry milk solids | 1 cup | 48 | 36 | |
| Ice water | 1 cup | | | |
| | | 74.4 | 53.4 | 6.4 |
| Calories: 1 serving—46.9 | | 6.2 | 4.4 | .5 |

Soften gelatin in water. Make paste of cocoa and milk. Heat over boiling water; add softened gelatin and artificial sweetener, stirring until gelatin dissolves. Remove from heat; add vanilla; and let stand until mixture thickens. Then combine milk solids and ice water; beat on high speed of mixer until of consistency of whipped cream. Beat gelatin smooth and gradually add to the whipped milk. Spoon into oiled 6-cup mold. Chill until firm, about 3 hours.

Servings: 12
Exchange per serving: 1 vegetable B

RECIPE FOR

# Cheese Pie

| Ingredients | Measure | Carbohydrates (gm.) | Protein (gm.) | Fat (gm.) |
|---|---|---|---|---|
| Low fat cream cheese | 16 ounces | 16.96 | 42.56 | 104.32 |
| Eggs | 3 | | 21 | 15 |
| Artificial sweetener, granulated | = ⅔ cup sugar | | | |
| Almond extract | ⅛ teaspoon | | | |
| Topping: | | | | |
| Sour cream | 1 pint | | | 90 |
| Artificial sweetener | = 3 tablespoons sugar | | | |
| Vanilla | 1 teaspoon | | | |
| | | 16.96 | 63.56 | 209.32 |
| Calories: 1 serving—221 | | 1.69 | 6.35 | 20.93 |

Beat cheese and add eggs, one at a time. Add artificial sweetener and extract and beat for 5 minutes. Pour into greased 9-inch pie pan. Bake at 325 degrees for 50 minutes. Cool 20 minutes. Spoon topping over top of pie. Bake 15 minutes. Cool and refrigerate.

You can also top the pie with can of sour cherries mixed well with 1 envelope cherry dietetic gelatin. Be sure to add ½ fruit exchange to each serving for the cherries.

Servings: 10
Exchange per serving: 1 meat, 3 fat

# Strawberry Whip

| Ingredients | Measure | Carbohydrates (gm.) | Protein (gm.) | Fat (gm.) |
|---|---|---|---|---|
| Strawberries, washed and hulled | 1 pint | 20 | | |
| Hot water | ½ cup | | | |
| Dietetic strawberry gelatin | 2 envelopes | | | |
| Crushed ice | 1¼ cups | | | |
| | | 20 | | |

Calories: 1 serving—10                    2.5

Wash and hull strawberries. Into an electric blender pour hot water, dry gelatin, and 1 cup of the strawberries. Cover; blend 30 seconds. Add crushed ice; blend 20 seconds longer. Add remaining strawberries. Blend about 3 seconds. Pour into chilled serving bowl. Chill 1 hour or until partially set. Spoon into serving dishes and garnish with mint, if desired.

Servings: 8
Exchange per serving: ¼ fruit

# Fruit Whip

| Ingredients | Measure | | Carbohydrates (gm.) | Protein (gm.) | Fat (gm.) |
|---|---|---|---|---|---|
| Fruit juice, unsweetened* | 1¾ | cups | 35 | | |
| Unflavored gelatin | 1 | envelope | | 7 | |
| Artificial sweetener | = 10 | teaspoons sugar | | | |
| Salt | ⅛ | teaspoon | | | |
| | | | 35 | 7 | |
| Calories: 1 serving—41.6 | | | 8.7 | 1.7 | |

Sprinkle gelatin over ½ cup fruit juice in saucepan. Cook over low heat, stirring constantly, until gelatin is dissolved. Remove from heat. Stir in artificial sweetener, salt, and remaining 1¼ cups fruit juice. Chill until thick but not set. Beat at highest speed until smooth and creamy. Chill until firm. Spoon into serving dishes.

*Orange, orange-grapefruit, apple, pineapple-orange, or pineapple-grapefruit.

Servings: 4
Exchange per serving: 1 vegetable B or 1 fruit

# Hawaiian Dessert

| Ingredients | Measure | | Carbohydrates (gm.) | Protein (gm.) | Fat (gm.) |
|---|---|---|---|---|---|
| Dietetic pineapple | 6 | slices | 60 | | |
| Reserved juice | ¾ | cup | | | |
| Dietetic lime gelatin | 2 | envelopes | | | |
| Milk, skim | ½ | cup | 6 | 4 | |
| Almond extract | ¼ | teaspoon | | | |
| Crushed ice | ¾ | cup | | | |
| | | | 66 | 4 | |
| Calories: 1 serving—46.4 | | | 11 | | .6 |

Bring juice to a boil; add gelatin, stirring until gelatin dissolves. Combine pineapple and milk in blender; blend well. Add gelatin mixture, almond extract, and ice. Mix thoroughly in blender. Pour into dessert dishes. Chill until set, about 1 hour.

Servings: 6
Exchange per serving: 1 fruit

# Baked Custard

| Ingredients | Measure | Car-bohy-drates (gm.) | Pro-tein (gm.) | Fat (gm.) |
|---|---|---|---|---|
| Egg, lightly beaten | 1 | | 7 | 5 |
| Artificial sweetener | = 3 teaspoons sugar | | | |
| Milk, skim | 1 cup | 12 | 8 | |
| Vanilla | ½ teaspoon | | | |
| Nutmeg | as desired | | | |
| | | 12 | 15 | 5 |
| Calories: 1 serving—76.5 | | 6 | 7.5 | 2.5 |

Combine beaten egg with artificial sweetener; slowly add skim milk and vanilla, blending well. Pour mixture equally into two custard cups;* top with a sprinkling of nutmeg. Bake in pan of hot water in moderate oven, 325 degrees, about 1 hour or until mixture does not adhere to knife.

*If you rinse cups in cold water before pouring in mixture, custard will not stick.

Servings: 2
Exchange per serving: ½ skim milk, ½ meat

# Jellied Blanc Mange

| Ingredients | Measure | Car- bohy- drates (gm.) | Pro- tein (gm.) | Fat (gm.) |
|---|---|---|---|---|
| Unflavored gelatin | 1 envelope | | | |
| Milk, skim | 2 cups | 24 | 16 | |
| Salt | ¼ teaspoon | | | |
| Extract | 1 teaspoon | | | |
| Artificial sweetener | = 8 teaspoons sugar | | | |
| | | 24 | 16 | |
| Calories: 1 serving—40 | | 6 | 4 | |

Soften gelatin in ¼ cup cold milk. Dissolve in 1¾ cups very hot milk. Add artificial sweetener, salt, and extract. Pour into 2-cup mold or 4 individual molds. Chill until firm, about 2 hours.

This recipe can be made with any flavor extract—rum, butterscotch, fruit extracts, vanilla, etc. Sprinkle nutmeg on top when using vanilla. It can be whipped after chilling until syrupy (yields 6 servings), or it can be whipped when set and layered with dietetic gelatin.

Servings: 4
Exchange per serving: ½ skim milk

# Eclairs

| Ingredients | Measure | Carbohy-drates (gm.) | Pro-tein (gm.) | Fat (gm.) |
|---|---|---|---|---|
| Water | ½ cup | | | |
| Margarine | 4 tablespoons | | | 60 |
| Flour, sifted | ½ cup | 38 | 5.4 | .4 |
| Salt | ⅛ teaspoon | | | |
| Eggs | 2 | | 14 | 10 |
| Dietetic vanilla pudding | 1 envelope | | | |
| Milk, skim | 1 cup | 12 | 8 | |
| | | 50 | 27.4 | 70.4 |
| Calories: 1 serving—188 | | 10 | 5.5 | 14 |

Heat water and margarine to boiling in medium saucepan. Stir in flour and salt all at once with a wooden spoon; continue stirring until batter forms a thick smooth ball that follows spoon around pan. Remove from heat; cool slightly; beat in eggs, one at a time, until mixture is thick and shiny-smooth. Shape batter into 5 strips on ungreased cookie sheet. Bake at 400 degrees for 30 minutes until puffed and lightly golden. Remove at once from cookie sheet and cool completely on wire rack. Prepare pudding mix with milk and chill. Cut slice across each eclair and lift off top. Scoop out softened dough. Fill with pudding. Replace top. Put teaspoon of dietetic chocolate syrup on top.

Servings: 5
Exchange per serving: 1 fruit, 1 meat, 2 fat

# Baked Alaska

| Ingredients | Measure | Carbohydrates (gm.) | Protein (gm.) | Fat (gm.) |
|---|---|---|---|---|
| Pound cake, 4x2¾x⅝ inches | 4 slices | 77.6 | 10 | 42.8 |
| Ice cream, any flavor | 1 pint | 60 | 8 | 40 |
| Egg whites | 3 | | .6 | 9.9 |
| Cream of tartar | ¼ teaspoon | | | |
| Salt | ⅛ teaspoon | | | |
| Artificial sweetener | = 6 tablespoons sugar | | | |
| Vanilla | ⅛ teaspoon | | | |
| | | 138.2 | 27.9 | 82.8 |
| Calories: 1 serving—351.9 | | 34.5 | 6.9 | 20.7 |

Place ½ cup ice cream in custard cup to mold and turn out on piece of cake. Repeat with remaining cake and ice cream and place in freezer for 15 minutes. Beat egg whites with cream of tartar and salt at very high speed until soft peaks form. Gradually beat in artificial sweetener; add vanilla. Continue beating until egg whites form stiff peaks. Remove ice cream and cake from freezer. Spread meringue over both. Completely seal with the meringue. Return to freezer. Place heavy brown paper on cookie sheet and grease well. Preheat oven to 425 degrees. Place frozen Alaskas on cookie sheet and bake 5 minutes, or until delicately browned. Serve at once.

Servings: 4

Exchange per serving: 2 bread, ⅓ milk, 3 fat, or 1 milk, 2 fruit, 2 fat

RECIPE FOR

# Pudding Surprise

| Ingredients | Measure | Carbohydrates (gm.) | Protein (gm.) | Fat (gm.) |
|---|---|---|---|---|
| Dietetic pudding, vanilla | 2 envelopes | | | |
| Milk, skim | 2 cups | 24 | 16 | |
| Dietetic jam, jelly, or marmalade | 8 teaspoons | | | |
| | | 24 | 16 | |

Calories: 1 serving—40      6  4

Prepare pudding according to package directions using skim milk. Rinse custard cups; place 2 teaspoons jam, jelly, or marmalade in each; pour in hot vanilla pudding; chill.

Servings: 4
Exchange per serving: ½ skim milk

# Frozen Dessert Shells

| Ingredients | Measure | Carbohydrates (gm.) | Protein (gm.) | Fat (gm.) |
|---|---|---|---|---|
| Dream Whip | 1 envelope | 19.2 | 9.6 | 19.2 |
| Cold milk, skim | ½ cup | 6 | 4 | |
| Vanilla | ½ teaspoon | | | |
| | | 25.2 | 13.6 | 19.2 |
| Calories: 1 serving—41 | | 3.15 | 1.7 | 2.4 |

Combine Dream Whip, milk, and vanilla and prepare as directed on package. Drop mixture onto wax paper, about ¼ cup at a time. With a spoon make a depression in the top of each mound. Freeze until firm, 2 to 3 hours. Fill shells just before serving.

Fillings:
1. ¼ cup fruit ice in each shell—add 1 fruit exchange
2. Cubes of dietetic gelatin—free
3. ¼ cup dietetic pudding—add ¼ milk exchange
4. ⅛ cup ice cream topped with dietetic chocolate syrup—add ¼ bread, ½ fat

Servings: 8
Exchange per serving: ½ vegetable B, ½ fat

# Bread Pudding

| Ingredients | Measure | | Carbohydrates (gm.) | Protein (gm.) | Fat (gm. |
|---|---|---|---|---|---|
| Bread, cubed | 2 | slices | 30 | 4 | |
| Eggs, slightly beaten | 2 | | | 14 | 10 |
| Artificial sweetener | = 16 | teaspoons sugar | | | |
| Vanilla | 1 | teaspoon | | | |
| Salt | ⅛ | teaspoon | | | |
| Milk, skim, scalded | 2 | cups | 24 | 16 | |
| Cinnamon | 1 | teaspoon | | | |
| | | | 54 | 34 | 10 |
| Calories: 1 serving—53.6 | | | 6.7 | 4 | 1.2 |

Place bread cubes in lightly greased 1-quart casserole. Combine eggs, artificial sweetener, vanilla, and salt and gradually add milk. Pour over bread cubes. Sprinkle with cinnamon. Place casserole in hot water in pan and bake at 325 degrees for 55 to 65 minutes.

Servings: 4
Exchange per serving: 1 vegetable B, ⅓ meat

# Parfait Royale

| Ingredients | Measure | | Car- bohy- drates (gm.) | Pro- tein (gm.) | Fat (gm.) |
|---|---|---|---|---|---|
| Dietetic apple-raspberry sauce | 15 | ounces | 52.5 | | |
| Dietetic vanilla pudding | 2 | envelopes | | | |
| Milk, skim | 2 | cups | 24 | 16 | |
| | | | 76.5 | 16 | |
| Calories: 1 serving—73.2 | | | 15.3 | 3 | |

Put 2 heaping tablespoons of sauce in each of 5 parfait glasses. Make pudding according to package directions and spoon evenly on top of sauce in parfait glasses. Let stand about 15 minutes until firm. Spoon remaining sauce on top of pudding. Refrigerate until chilled.

Servings: 5
Exchange per serving: 1 fruit, ½ skim milk

CHAPTER XVIII

# Cakes

# Cakes

# Spiced Cake

| Ingredients | Measure | Carbohydrates (gm.) | Protein (gm.) | Fat (gm.) |
|---|---|---|---|---|
| Margarine | ½ cup | | | 120 |
| Artificial sweetener | = ¼ cup sugar | | | |
| Eggs | 2 | | 14 | 10 |
| Skim sour milk | 1 cup | 12 | 8 | |
| Vanilla | 1 teaspoon | | | |
| Flour | 2 cups | 151.8 | 21.6 | 1.8 |
| Cinnamon | 2 teaspoons | | | |
| Cloves | ½ teaspoon | | | |
| Alspice | 2 teaspoons | | | |
| Nutmeg | 1 teaspoon | | | |
| Baking soda | 1 teaspoon | | | |
| | | 163.8 | 43.6 | 131.8 |

Calories: 1 serving—125.4          10.2    2.7    8.2

Cream margarine with artificial sweetener. Add eggs. Combine dry ingredients. Add milk alternately with dry ingredients. Add vanilla. Pour into 8x8x2-inch pan. Bake at 350 degrees for 30 minutes. Cut into sixteen 2-inch pieces.

Servings: 16
Exchange per serving: 1 vegetable B, 1½ fat

# Coffee Crumb Cakes

| Ingredients | Measure | | Carbohydrates (gm.) | Protein (gm.) | Fat (gm.) |
|---|---|---|---|---|---|
| Flour | 2 | cups | 151.8 | 21.6 | 1.8 |
| Double-acting baking powder | 3 | teaspoons | | | |
| Salt | ¾ | teaspoon | | | |
| Cinnamon | ¼ | teaspoon | | | |
| Baking soda | ¼ | teaspoon | | | |
| Nutmeg | ¼ | teaspoon | | | |
| Margarine | ½ | cup | | | 120 |
| Milk, skim | 1 | cup | 12 | 8 | |
| Instant coffee | ¼ | teaspoon | | | |
| Egg, unbeaten | 1 | | | 7 | 5 |
| Artificial sweetener | = ½ | cup sugar | | | |
| | | | 163.8 | 36.6 | 126.8 |

Calories: 1 serving—107      9    2    7

Sift together flour, baking powder, salt, cinnamon, baking soda, and nutmeg. Cut in margarine until particles are fine. Reserve scant ¼ cup for topping. Combine milk, coffee, egg, and artificial sweetener. Add all at once to remaining crumb mixture. Stir 100 strokes with a spoon. Fill 18 muffin cups, lined with paper baking cups, half full. Sprinkle with reserved crumb topping. Bake at 375 degrees for 20 to 25 minutes.

Servings: 18
Exchange per serving: ½ bread, 1 fat

# Sponge Cupcakes

| Ingredients | Measure | Carbohydrates (gm.) | Protein (gm.) | Fat (gm.) |
|---|---|---|---|---|
| Eggs, separated | 3 | | 21 | 15 |
| Salt | ¼ teaspoon | | | |
| Cream of tartar | ¼ teaspoon | | | |
| Artificial sweetener | = 8 teaspoons sugar | | | |
| Lemon juice | 1 teaspoon | | | |
| Lemon rind | few gratings | | | |
| Flour, sifted | ½ cup | 38 | 5.4 | .4 |
| | | 38 | 26.4 | 15.4 |
| Calories: 1 serving—39.1 | | 3.8 | 2.6 | 1.5 |

Add salt to egg whites and beat until foamy. Add cream of tartar and continue beating until stiff, but not dry. Beat egg yolks until thick. Add artificial sweetener, lemon juice, and lemon rind while continuing to beat. Quickly and carefully fold egg yolks and flour which has been sifted several times into egg whites. Drop by spoonfuls into greased muffin pans or waxed paper baking cups. Bake at 350 degrees for 18 minutes.

Servings: 10
Exchange per serving: ⅓ skim milk, ⅓ fat

# Low Sugar Cupcakes

| Ingredients | Measure | Carbohydrates (gm.) | Protein (gm.) | Fat (gm.) |
|---|---|---|---|---|
| Margarine | 6 tablespoons | | | 90 |
| Egg | 1 | | 7 | 5 |
| Milk, skim | ½ cup | 6 | 4 | |
| Flour | 1⅓ cups | 101.2 | 14.4 | 1.2 |
| Vanilla | ⅔ teaspoon | | | |
| Baking powder | 3 teaspoons | | | |
| Artificial sweetener granulated | = ½ cup sugar | | | |
| | | 107.2 | 25.4 | 96.2 |

Calories: 1 serving—116      8.9    2.1    8

Cream margarine; add artificial sweetener and egg. Combine milk and vanilla. Sift together flour and baking powder. Add flour and milk mixtures alternately to margarine mixture. Spoon into 12 small muffin cups. Bake at 350 degrees for 25 to 30 minutes.

Servings: 12
Exchange per serving: 1 vegetable B, 1½ fat

# Aunt Tillie's Favorite Brownie Recipe

| Ingredients | Measure | Carbohydrates (gm.) | Protein (gm.) | Fat (gm.) |
|---|---|---|---|---|
| Chocolate, semi-sweet | 4 ounces | 73.2 | 5.6 | 31.6 |
| Milk, skim | ½ cup | 6 | 4 | |
| Shortening | 1 cup | | | 240 |
| Artificial sweetener, granulated | = 2 cups sugar | | | |
| Eggs | 4 | | 28 | 20 |
| Flour | 1½ cups | 113.8 | 16.2 | 1.3 |
| Salt | ½ teaspoon | | | |
| Baking powder | 1 teaspoon | | | |
| Vanilla | 1 teaspoon | | | |
| | | 193 | 53.8 | 292.9 |
| Calories: 1 serving—92.7 | | 5 | 1.3 | 7.5 |

Melt chocolate in milk and let cool. Cream shortening; add artificial sweetener and eggs. Add chocolate mixture, dry ingredients, vanilla. Bake in greased 13x9x2-inch pan at 350 degrees for 30 minutes or until toothpick comes out dry when checked. Cut brownies when cool into 39 pieces, 3x1-inch.

If desired, add ½ cup chopped walnuts to batter or sprinkle on top before baking. This will then give ½ bread and 2 fat exchanges per brownie.

Servings: 39
Exchange per serving: ½ bread, 1½ fat

# Breakfast Coffee Cake

| Ingredients | Measure | Car-bohy-drates (gm.) | Pro-tein (gm.) | Fat (gm.) |
|---|---|---|---|---|
| Milk, skim | ¼ cup | 3 | 2 | |
| Margarine | ⅓ cup | | | 79.5 |
| Salt | 1 teaspoon | | | |
| Artificial sweetener | = 12 teaspoons sugar | | | |
| Yeast | 2 packages | | | |
| Water, lukewarm | ½ cup | | | |
| Eggs, beaten | 2 | | 14 | 10 |
| Flour | 3 cups | 227.7 | 3.2 | 2.7 |
| Walnuts, chopped | ⅓ cup | | | 25 |
| | | 230.7 | 19.2 | 117.2 |
| Calories: 1 serving—227.8 | | 25.6 | 2.1 | 13 |

Scald milk; add margarine, salt, and artificial sweetener; stir until margarine is melted. Cool to lukewarm. Dissolve yeast in warm water; add to the milk mixture. Add beaten eggs and flour, mix well and spoon into a greased 9-inch-square cake pan. Let rise, covered, in warm place until double in bulk. Scatter the chopped walnuts over top with light sprinkling of granulated artificial sweetener and cinnamon. Bake at 400 degrees for 20 minutes.

Servings: 9
Exchange per serving: 1 bread, 1 fruit, 2½ fat

# CHAPTER XIX

# Cookies

NABISCO COOKIES:

| | |
|---|---|
| 5 vanilla wafers | 1 bread |
| 3 lemon snaps | 1 bread |
| 3 brown edge wafers | 1 bread |
| 3 arrowroot | 1 bread |
| 3 ginger snaps | 1 bread |
| 5 animal crackers | 1 bread |
| 3 chocolate snaps | 1 bread |
| 3 butter thins | 1 bread |
| 2 oreos | 1 bread |
| 1½ fig newtons | 1 bread |
| 2 chocolate grahams | 1 bread, 1 fat |

Toll House Cookies—made by recipe on Nestle's chocolate chip package
    12 ounce package—100 cookies

| | |
|---|---|
| 2 cookies | 1 bread |

There are very few *good* diabetic cookie recipes and even the few in this manual are best when fresh. I prefer to use commercial cookies sparingly.

# Smackaroons

| Ingredients | Measure | | Carbohydrates (gm.) | Protein (gm.) | Fat (gm.) |
|---|---|---|---|---|---|
| Egg whites | 3 | | | .6 | 9.9 |
| Double-acting baking powder | ½ | teaspoon | | | |
| Flour | 2 | tablespoons | 22.4 | 3 | |
| Artificial sweetener | = 16 | teaspoons sugar | | | |
| Almond extract | ½ | teaspoon | | | |
| Rice crispy cereal | 2½ | cups | 50 | 6.7 | |
| Coconut, unsweetened | ¼ | cup | 12 | 3.6 | 32.4 |
| | | | 85 | 23.2 | 32.4 |
| Calories: 4 cookies—118.8 | | | 14 | 4 | 5.2 |

Beat egg whites with baking powder until stiff but not dry. Blend in flour, artificial sweetener, almond extract, cereal, and coconut. Drop by rounded teaspoonfuls onto lightly greased cookie sheets. Bake at 350 degrees for 12 minutes.

Servings: 24 cookies
Exchange per serving: 4 cookies—1 bread, 1 fat

# Cinnamon Cookies

| Ingredients | Measure | Carbohydrates (gm.) | Protein (gm.) | Fat (gm.) |
|---|---|---|---|---|
| Margarine | 5 tablespoons | | | 75 |
| Flour | 1 cup | 75.9 | 10.8 | .3 |
| Baking powder | ½ teaspoon | | | |
| Cinnamon | 1 teaspoon | | | |
| Salt | pinch | | | |
| Artificial sweetener | = 16 teaspoons sugar | | | |
| Vanilla | 1 teaspoon | | | |
| Milk | 1 tablespoon | .7 | .5 | .6 |
| | | 76.6 | 11.3 | 75.9 |
| Calories: 4 cookies—134.8 | | 10 | 1.2 | 10 |

Cream margarine, blend in flour, baking powder, cinnamon, and salt. Mix artificial sweetener with vanilla and milk. Stir into flour mixture and mix thoroughly. Shape dough into 30 balls and place on cookie sheet. Flatten balls with fork dipped in cold water. Bake at 375 degrees for 15 minutes.

Servings: 30 cookies

Exchange per serving: 4 cookies—1 fruit, 2 fat

RECIPE FOR

# Pinwheel Cookies

| Ingredients | Measure | Car-bohy-drates (gm.) | Pro-tein (gm.) | Fat (gm.) |
|---|---|---|---|---|
| Flour | 1½ cups | 113.8 | 16.2 | 1.3 |
| Shortening | ½ cup | | | 120 |
| Orange juice | ¼ cup | 5 | | |
| Margarine, soft | 2 tablespoons | | | 30 |
| Nuts, chopped | ⅓ cup | | | 25 |
| | | 118.8 | 16.2 | 176.3 |
| Calories: 1 cookie—34.5 | | 1.9 | .2 | 2.9 |

Cut shortening into flour. Add juice and mix well. Divide into three portions and roll out each piece. Spread with soft margarine and sprinkle with mixture of nuts, cinnamon, and powdered artificial sweetener to taste. Roll and slice ¼ inch. Place cookies on sheet and bake at 450 degrees for 12 minutes.

The cookies can be spread with dietetic jelly instead of nut, cinnamon, and sugar mixture. In that case omit softened margarine. This will make each cookie 2 grams of fat instead of 2.9.

Servings: 60
Exchange per serving: ⅛ bread, ½ fat

# Chapter XX

# Beverages

| | |
|---|---|
| Nestle's cocoa—3 heaping teaspoons | 1 bread |
| Chocolate Quik— | |
| 2 heaping teaspoons | 1½ fruit |
| Strawberry Quik— | |
| 2 heaping teaspoons | 1½ fruit |
| Nestle's Quik Shake—1-ounce | 1 bread, 1 fruit |
| | *or* 2½ fruit |
| Malted milk powder—1 tablespoon | ½ bread |
| Great Shakes—1 envelope | 1 bread, 1 fruit |

Be sure to count the milk used in any of the above beverages; the values given are for the powders alone.

A special note regarding diet sodas: With the recent ban on cyclamates, many manufacturers were forced to add sugar to their products to provide a pleasing taste. The diet sodas are still lower in calories than the regular ones, but the diabetic, who had been able to drink a bottle as a "free" food, now finds that six-ounces must be counted as a fruit exchange.

# Tomato Tantalizer

| Ingredients | Measure | | Carbohydrates (gm.) | Protein (gm.) | Fat (gm.) |
|---|---|---|---|---|---|
| Tomato juice | 20 | ounces | | | |
| Instant minced onion | 1 | tablespoon | | | |
| Artificial sweetener | = ½ | teaspoon sugar | | | |
| Salt | ½ | teaspoon | | | |
| Worcestershire sauce | ¼ | teaspoon | | | |
| Tabasco | | dash | | | |

Combine all ingredients. Refrigerate. Serve in pre-chilled glasses. Sprinkle with coarse ground pepper.

Servings: 4
Exchange per serving: free

# Ice Cream Float

| Ingredients | Measure | Carbohydrates (gm.) | Protein (gm.) | Fat (gm.) |
|---|---|---|---|---|
| Vanilla ice cream | ½ cup | 15 | 2 | 10 |
| Noncaloric carbonated beverage | 8 ounces | | | |
| Calories: 1 serving—158 | | 15 | 2 | 10 |

Put ice cream in glass and pour beverage on top.

Servings: 1
Exchange per serving: 1 bread, 2 fat

# Milkshake

| Ingredients | Measure | Car-bohy-drates (gm.) | Pro-tein (gm.) | Fat (gm.) |
|---|---|---|---|---|
| Milk, skim | ½ cup | 6 | 4 | |
| Artificial sweetener | = ½ teaspoon sugar | | | |
| Ice cube | 1 | | | |
| Vanilla | ⅛ teaspoon | | | |
| Calories: 1 serving—40 | | 6 | 4 | |

Place all ingredients in electric blender and blend until milkshake foams up and ice cube disappears.

In place of vanilla you can use almost any extract that pleases you—banana, orange, peppermint, etc.

Servings: 1
Exchange per serving: ½ skim milk

# Appendix

| | Carbo-hydrate (gm.) | Pro-tein (gm.) | Fat (gm.) | Calories |
|---|---|---|---|---|
| White commercial flour | | | | |
| 1 cup | 75.9 | 10.8 | .9 | 354.9 |
| ½ cup | 37.9 | 5.4 | .4 | 176.8 |
| 1 tablespoon | 11.2 | 1.5 | | 50.8 |
| Orange juice frozen concentrate | | | | |
| 1 ounce | 10 | | | 40. |
| Unflavored gelatin—1 envelope | | 7 | | 28 |
| Graham crackers | | | | |
| 1 cup, crushed (12 crackers) | 90 | 12 | | 408 |
| Tomato sauce—2 ounces | 7 | 2 | | 36 |
| Tomato paste—1 ounce | 7 | 2 | | 36 |
| Ground meat—raw | | | | |
| 1 pound | | 84 | 60 | 876 |
| ½ pound | | 42 | 30 | 438 |
| ¼ pound | | 21 | 15 | 219 |
| Corn starch—2 tablespoons | 15 | 2 | | 68 |
| Uncooked macaroni—1 ounce | 15 | 2 | | 68 |
| Catsup—1 tablespoon | 4.9 | .4 | | 21.2 |
| Brown sugar—1 tablespoon | 13 | | | 52 |
| Marshmallows—8 | 6.5 | .2 | | 26.8 |
| 1 ounce | 23 | 1 | | 96 |
| Johnston's graham cracker crust | | | | |
| whole | 117 | 9.1 | 36 | 828.4 |
| ⅛ pie crust | 15 | 1.1 | 4.5 | 104.9 |
| Johnston's chocolate crust | | | | |
| whole | 107 | 8.8 | 38 | 805.2 |
| ⅛ pie crust | 13 | 1.1 | 4.7 | 98.7 |
| Baker's Chocolate | | | | |
| German Sweet— | | | | |
| 4½ square—1-ounce | 16.6 | 1.1 | 10.2 | 162.6 |

| | Carbo-hydrate (gm.) | Pro-tein (gm.) | Fat (gm.) | Calories |
|---|---|---|---|---|
| Semi-sweet chips— | | | | |
| 1 square—1 ounce | | | | |
| 1/16 cup—1-ounce | 18.3 | 1.4 | 7.9 | 147.9 |
| Unsweetened—1 square—1-ounce | 8 | 4 | 15.1 | 183.9 |
| Dream Whip—1 tablespoon | .6 | .3 | .6 | 9 |
| Unsweetened coconut—¼ cup | 12 | 3.6 | 32.4 | 354 |
| Bisquick—1 cup | 76 | 9.5 | 14.5 | 472.5 |
| Whip'n Chill (made with all water) | | | | |
| (yields 5 servings) ½ cup | 15 | 3 | 3 | 87 |
| Walnuts, chopped ⅓ cup | | | 25 | 225 |

## FROZEN MEALS

MORTON:

| | |
|---|---|
| Chicken pot pie | 2½ bread, 2 meat, 3 fat |
| Turkey pot pie | 2½ bread, 2 meat, 3 fat |
| Ham dinner | 3½ bread, 2 meat |
| Turkey dinner | 1½ bread, 4 meat |
| Shrimp dinner | 2 bread, 2 meat, 1½ fat |
| Beef dinner | 1½ bread, 4 meat |
| Salisbury steak dinner | 1 bread, 4 meat, 1 fat |
| Meat loaf dinner | 1½ bread, 3 meat, 2 fat |
| Fish dinner | 2 bread, 3 meat |
| Fried chicken dinner | 1½ bread, 4 meat, ½ fat |

SWANSON:

| | |
|---|---|
| Turkey meat pie (8-ounce) | 2 meat, 2½ bread, 3 fat |
| Chicken meat pie (8-ounce) | 2 meat, 1 fruit, 1 bread, 3 fat |
| Beef meat pie (8-ounce) | 2 meat, 2½ bread, 3 fat |
| Tuna pie (8-ounce) | 2 meat, 2½ bread, 3 fat |
| Chicken deep dish pie (1 pound) | 4 meat, 1½ bread, 1 fruit, 4 fat |
| Beef deep dish pie (1 pound) | 5 meat, 1 bread, 1 fruit, 2 fat |

| | |
|---|---|
| Turkey deep dish pie (1 pound) | 4 meat, 1 bread, 1 fruit, 2 fat |
| Turkey 3 course dinner | 4 meat, 1 bread, 1 fruit |
| Salisbury steak 3 course dinner | 4 meat, 1 bread, 1 fruit |
| Beef 3 course dinner | 4 meat, 1 fruit, 1 bread |
| Fried chicken 3 course dinner | 4 meat, 1 bread, 2 fruit |
| Mixed seafood grill 3 course dinner | 3 meat, 1 bread, 1 fruit |

## CANDY

| | |
|---|---|
| 6 Hershey kisses | 1 bread, 1 fat |
| 35 M & M's | 1 bread, 1½ fat |
| 1-ounce Nestle's milk chocolate | 1 bread, 2 fat |
| 1-ounce Nestle's almond | 1 bread, 2 fat |
| 1-ounce Nestle's crunch | 1 bread, 1½ fat |
| 10 jelly beans | 1 bread |
| Mars or Milky Way, 1¼-ounce | 2 bread |
| Snickers, 1¼-ounce | 1⅔ bread |
| Forever Yours, 1¼-ounce | 1⅔ bread |
| Three Musketeers, 1⅜-ounce | 2⅓ bread |
| Lollipop, ½-ounce | 1 bread |
| Gumdrops, 2 (⅞-inch diameter) | 1 bread |
| 12 small | 1 bread |
| Kraft caramels, 2 | 1 bread |
| Life savers 6 | 1 bread |
| 4 | 1 fruit |

# Weights and Measures

| | |
|---|---|
| 1 teaspoon | ⅓ tablespoon |
| 1 tablespoon | 3 teaspoons |
| ¼ cup | 4 tablespoons |
| ⅓ cup | 5⅓ tablespoons |
| 1 cup (liquid)—8-ounces | 16 tablespoons |
| 1 ounce (liquid) | 2 tablespoons |
| 1 ounce (dry measure) | 1/16 pound |
| 1 pint | 2 cups |
| 1 quart | 2 pints |

| 1 gallon | 4 quarts |
|----------|----------|
| 1 gill | ½ cup |
| 1 bushel | 4 pecks |

# How to Calculate Favorite Recipes

On a blank sheet list each ingredient, the amount to be used for the recipe, and the carbohydrate, protein, and fat of this amount in grams in the proper columns. (This can be found for most items in the beginning of each exchange category or in the listing of products in the Appendix.)

Add up the totals in each column and divide by the number of servings. This will tell you the amount of carbohydrate, protein, and fat for each serving. Using the chart below, calculate how many of each exchange the serving will cover.

Figures are in grams per exchange

| | Carbo-hydrate | Pro-tein | Fat | Calories |
|-----------|------|-----|-----|----------|
| Milk | 12 | 8 | 10 | 170 |
| Vegetable A | | | | |
| Vegetable B | 7 | 2 | | 36 |
| Fruit | 10 | | | 40 |
| Bread | 15 | 2 | | 68 |
| Meat | | 7 | 5 | 73 |
| Fat | | | 5 | 45 |

# Bibliography

Campbell Soup Company
Camden, New Jersey
List of Campbell, Red Kettle and Bounty products and their exchanges (free)

Department of Nutrition
National Live Stock and Meat Board
407 South Dearborn Street
Chicago, Illinois
Nutrition Yardstick

General Foods Kitchens
250 North Street
White Plains, New York 10602
List of Baker's, Bird's Eye and other products with carbohydrate, fat and protein values per serving (free)

H. J. Heinz Company
Pittsburgh, Pennsylvania
List of Heinz products and their exchanges (free)

Superintendent of Documents
U.S. Government Printing Office
Washington, D. C. 20402
United States Department of Agriculture Handbook #8 *Composition of Foods* ($1.50)

## VALUABLE REFERENCE SOURCES

Eli Lilly and Company
Public Relations Services
Indianapolis, Indiana 46206
*A Guide for the Diabetic* (free)

Ames Company
Division Miles Laboratories, Inc.
1127 Myrtle Street
Elkhart, Indiana 46514
*Guidebook for the Diabetic Patient* (free)

*In Diabetes Good Timing Goes Hand in Hand with Good Control* (free)
*Diabetes in the Middle Years* (free)

Professional and Guest Relations
(Unit 9250)
Upjohn Company
Kalamazoo, Michigan 49001
*You and Diabetes* (free)
*How to Live with Diabetes* (free)

Pfizer Laboratories
Brooklyn, New York
*If You Have Diabetes* (free)

Public Health Service Publications: (single copy free)

Inquiry Branch
Health Services & Mental Health Administration
U.S. Dept. of Health, Education and Welfare
Washington, D. C. 20201
*Six Food Exchange Lists* (#326)
*Diabetes and You* (#567)
*Foot Care for the Diabetic Patient* (#1153)
*Diabetes* (#137)
*Answers to Questions That Are Often Asked About Diabetic Diets* (#1847)
    Multiple copies of the above pamphlets may be ordered from:
        Superintendent of Documents
        U.S. Government Printing Office
        Washington, D. C. 20402
            #567 —25¢
            #1153— 5¢ ($3/100)
            #326 — 5¢ ($3/100)
            #137 — 5¢ ($2.50/100)
            #1847—10¢ ($6.75/100)

American Diabetes Assoc., Inc.
18 East 48th Street
New York, New York 10017
*Meal Planning with Exchange Lists* (free)

Good Housekeeping Bulletin Service
959 Eighth Avenue
New York, New York 10019
*Good Housekeeping's Cookbook for Diabetics* (50¢)
    125 recipes with exchanges
*Good Housekeeping's Diets for Diabetics* (50¢)
    Menu suggestions and recipes with exchanges

Knox Gelatin, Incorporated
Johnstown, New York 12095
*New Variety in Meal Planning for the Diabetic* (free)
    Recipes with diabetic exchanges

Education for Health, Inc.
510 Plymouth Avenue
Minneapolis, Minnesota 55411
*Diabetic Cooking Made Easy* by Virginia M. Donahoe ($1.)

University of Texas Press
Post Office Box 7819
Austin, Texas 78712
*The Diabetic's Cookbook* by Elsie B. Strachan ($2.95)

Taplinger Publishing Company, Inc.
29 East 10th Street
New York, New York 10003
*Cookbook for Diabetics* by Gaynor Maddox ($1.95)

Hawthorn Books, Incorporated
70 Fifth Avenue
New York, New York 10011
*The Peripatetic Diabetic* by Margaret Bennett ($5.95)

*Better Homes and Gardens*
Meredith Press
1716 Locust Street
Des Moines, Iowa 50303
*Eat and Stay Slim* ($1.95)
    A diet plan based on the diabetic exchange system with recipes giving
    exchanges in a color-coded system.

Frederick Fell, Incorporated
386 Park Avenue South
New York, New York 10016
*Food Values and Calorie Charts* by Jules G. Szanton
Breakdown of brand name foods giving carbohydrate, protein, and fat values as well as other tables. ($2.95 plus 25¢ for postage and handling)

## CHILDREN

Ames Company
Division Miles Laboratories, Inc.
1127 Myrtle Street
Elkhart, Indiana 46514
*Mr. Hypo is My Friend* (free)

Greater Boston Diabetes Society, Inc.
93 Massachusetts Avenue
Boston, Massachusetts 02115
3 *Wheels Coloring Book* by Catherine McQuaid (50¢)
Coloring book especially for diabetic children

Frederick Fell, Incorporated
386 Park Avenue South
New York, New York 10016
*The Care and Feeding of Your Diabetic Child* by Sally Vanderpoel ($4.95 plus 25¢ for postage and handling)

## HANDBOOKS

The Diabetes Press of America
30 Southeast Eighth Street
Miami, Florida 33131
*Diabetes for Diabetics* by George G. Schmitt, M.D. ($6.95)

Doubleday and Company
501 Franklin Avenue
Garden City, New York 11530
Att: Mr. Arthur Parsons
*The New Way to Live with Diabetes* by Charles Weller, M.D. and Brian Richard Boyles ($3.95)

American Diabetes Assoc., Inc.
8 East 48th Street
New York, New York 10017
*Forecast Magazine* ($3. per year)

Education for Health, Inc.
510 Plymouth Avenue
Minneapolis, Minnesota 55411
*The Diabetic* ($1 per year 4 issues)

*Diabetes in the News*
Post Office Box 906
Elkhart, Indiana 46514
*Diabetes in the News* ($1 per year)

## PROGRAMMED TEACHING COURSE

South Texas Diabetes Assoc., Inc.
P.O. Box 2577
Texas City, Texas 77590
*An Instructional Aid on Juvenile Diabetes Mellitus* by Luther B. Travis, M.D. ($1.50)

## MISCELLANEOUS

Diabetes Assoc. of Greater Cleveland
2980 Mayfield Road
Cleveland Heights, Ohio 44118
Instant glucose (4 tubes for $1.)

The Diabetes Press of America
30 Southeast Eighth Street
Miami, Florida 33131
*Teaching Slides for Diabetics* ($60.)
    203 slides:
        The Pancreas
        Identification Insignia
        Measuring Equipment
        The Exchange Lists
        Insulin
        Glucagon
        Urine Testing

## DATE DUE

| | | | |
|---|---|---|---|
| | | | |
| | | | |
| | | | |
| | | | |
| | | | |
| | | | |
| | | | |
| | | | |
| | | | |
| | | | |
| | | | |
| | | | |
| | | | |
| | | | |
| | | | |
| | | | |
| | | | |
| | | | |
| GAYLORD | | | PRINTED IN U.S.A. |